Zen Shiatsu

D1033785

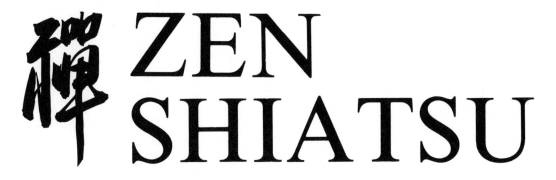

ZEN SHIATSU

How to Harmonize Yin and Yang for Better Health

By **Shizuto Masunaga**
with **Wataru Ohashi**

and the Shiatsu Education Center of America

Japan Publications, Inc.

© 1977 by Japan Publications, Inc.

Published by
JAPAN PUBLICATIONS, INC., Tokyo and New York

Distributors:
UNITED STATES: *Kodansha America, Inc., through Farrar, Straus & Giroux, 19 Union Square West, New York, N.Y. 10003.* CANADA: *Fitzhenry & Whiteside Ltd., 195 Allstate Parkway, Markham, Ontario L3R 4T8.* BRITISH ISLES AND EUROPEAN CONTINENT: *Premier Book Marketing Ltd., 1 Gower Street, London WC1E 6HA.* AUSTRALIA AND NEW ZEALAND: *Bookwise International, 54 Crittenden Road, Findon, South Australia 5023.* THE FAR EAST AND JAPAN: *Japan Publications Trading Co., Ltd., 1–2–1, Sarugaku-cho, Chiyoda-ku, Tokyo 101.*

First edition: September 1977
Fifteenth printing: December 1994

ISBN 0–87040–394–X
LCCC No. 77–74653

Printed in U.S.A.

Preface

There are many aspects of Japanese culture that have been influenced by Zen: kendo, archery, judo, Japanese gardening, architecture, tea ceremony, flower arrangement, Noh, brush painting, calligraphy, haiku, and even cooking with such foods as *tofu*, fermented soybeans, salted plums, *miso* soup, etc. In fact its influence is so common that most Japanese have forgotten its importance. Most Japanese believe that Zen is only one of the religious sects of Buddhism or simply training through meditation to be a monk. However, with the popularity of Zen in the West, many Japanese are taking a second look at Zen to rediscover oriental wisdom in relation to the culture, health, and way of life.

The fundamental purpose of Zen is to achieve total human enlightenment through the discovery of one's self.

Shiatsu is a form of physical manipulation that was developed in Japan in the twentieth century. Its origin comes from ancient Chinese techniques, *Do-In* and *anma*. Do-In is very similar to yoga while anma resembles western massage. These two techniques are the oldest forms of medical treatment in the Orient.

In modern times, modern manipulative therapy like chiropractic and osteopathy mainly imported from America, established a new status in medicine. Massage was still considered as a more or less medical substitute. In Japan, anma is practiced mainly by the blind for the purpose of pleasure and comfort. It wasn't until recently that authentic shiatsu came into being for the sole purpose of medical treatment. In order to distinguish shiatsu from anma, shiatsu therapists intentionally borrowed western medical theory to explain this particular type of treatment. Some therapists blindly emphasized that only pressing can cure all diseases. This same attitude also governs those who think that only sitting meditation in Zen will achieve *satori*. Unfortunately this attitude passes over any profound meanings behind it. It is true that Zen begins with meditation but it is not clear why we sit to meditate. Because answers in Zen cannot be thought out by the brain, there is a chance that understanding can be achieved through meditation.

The same with shiatsu. It begins with pressure with the fingers but it is difficult to explain why pressing the point cures disease. In both Zen and shiatsu we are dealing with something that cannot be explained rationally but that should be felt by the living body.

In Zen it is difficult to grasp and comprehend the wisdom behind oriental philosophy, but this is necessary in order to understand what Zen is all about. In shiatsu, simply pressing will not reveal to you the life essence of what you are pressing. Without knowledge of oriental philosophy you will not be able to comprehend the meaning of life and therefore administer shiatsu incorrectly. I published a book a while back to explain and show the effectiveness of shiatsu based on oriental medical theory. The underlying principle I stressed was, like Zen, to establish a life "echo" with the receiver of shiatsu. Some Japanese are satisfied with not noticing this important feeling, but this reduces shiatsu to a mechanical technique rather than a means of healing the life force within our bodies.

In Zen it is important that you have a good master to learn from. In shiatsu your patient is your master. You can achieve *satori* by curing diseases and restoring health. Most important is that you diagnose by touching. In Japanese we call this type of diagnosis *setsu-shin*. In this type of diagnosis we are not looking for a particular disease. Rather we are trying to understand the patient psychologically as well as physically. My method has been explained in the Japanese book, *Zen Treatment*, edited by Professor Koji Sato who is a psychologist and also my teacher from high school days. He also devoted his life to disseminating the principles of Zen overseas. The basic philosophy of this book comes from Hakuin Zenshi who emphasized self-anma. Professor Sato maintains that shiatsu for the patient is a kind of mutually man to man Zen. Deshimaru Roshi in Paris studied shiatsu with an introduction from Professor Sato. He used shiatsu on one of his students to correct the alignment of the spine. He not only corrected the spine but also cured diseases.

There are several schools of shiatsu but it is difficult to find a shiatsu practitioner practicing shiatsu based on the theory of oriental medicine. Most shiatsu techniques introduced in the West are for home remedy rather than treatment.

It is believed that oriental medicine was largely influenced by Indian medicine. When I was reading a Buddhist sutra, the zo-agonkyo, which is practiced in India, one passage was caught by my eye. It explained how the royal king of medicine should know the disease well, find its origin and cause, treat the disease, and care for and enlighten himself as to the constitution of his being. This to me is the ideal attitude toward medicine. Confucius in China states that he is the pivot whose function is to connect heaven, earth, and humans. This means that he plays a major role in combining the universal order of nature and morals of mankind. This is not an attitude of arrogance but awareness of himself in relation to universal rule. We who are dealing with medicine should aim for the same goal.

With this in mind, I established the Royal Medicine Institute in Tokyo where research and studies have been going on for more than 15 years. I have been intending to disseminate this knowledge to laymen as well as to professionals.

Oriental medicine is not as rational as western medicine but if we respect the mysteries of life and make the patient aware of himself, disease will disappear and the patient will endeavor to get well on his own. By applying your hand on a point or *tsubo* and following the meridian lines with your fingers, you may feel the "echo" of life. If you can receive and understand this sensation, disease will seem to disappear.

In writing this book I hope to explain the techniques not only from a mechanical point of view but from a philosophical aspect that will enable you to understand the essence of what you are doing. I believe that it is not our right but our duty to be healthy.

SHIZUTO MASUNAGA

Contents

1. Zen Shiatsu Philosophy

The History of Shiatsu in Japan

Recognition of shiatsu in Japan as a bona fide type of manipulative therapy came about 70 years ago and has been popular among the public for about 50 years. Government regulations were first issued for anma or Japanese massage practitioners requiring that they should be licensed in order to practice.

To avoid these regulations many therapists already in practice changed the name of their type of treatment. Thus the term *shiatsu* came into being. As this form of treatment became popular due to its simple but effective techniques, it was recognized as a legitimate form of therapy.

The three legally recognized forms of manipulative therapy in Japan are anma, western massage, and shiatsu. Some professional therapists insist that a great difference exists among the three forms of treatment. I believe that great differences cannot exist within one general field, in this case, manually applied stimulation to the human body. Of course, there are a variety of methods and schools, but basically they are similar. In Japan people refer to shiatsu as a form of medical treatment and distinguish it from anma in this way. The reasoning behind this is not because of the techniques involved but because anma was considered more for pleasure than health and was performed by the blind.

It is important to note that effectiveness of any treatment depends on both the practitioner and method working together. So the effectiveness of any treatment can vary greatly from one practitioner to another.

The Effectiveness of Different Forms of Treatment

In ancient standard textbooks on anma, the anma method described consisted of diagnosis and treatment. This was the first whole approach toward medicine. About 1,000 years ago Chinese medicine was introduced into Japan. At that time, the anma method was well-known in the medical field and was considered the safest and easiest method to treat the human body. During the Edo era (about 300 years ago) doctors in Japan were required to study anma in order to understand and become familiar with the structure of the human body and its functioning in terms of the meridian lines. Their training in this type of manual therapy enabled them to accurately diagnose and administer Chinese herbal medicine as well as locate the tsubos, which are the so-called acupuncture points, easily for acupuncture treatments when they became independent.

Unfortunately this ancient manipulation method was reduced to treating only simple problems like frozen shoulders and back tension and referred to as a blind man's profession. Because blind people were at a disadvantage in receiving formal study in diagnosis and treatment, anma gradually became associated with pleasure and comfort.

Western massage as an ancient form of manipulation is documented in Egyptian and Greek history. It is recognized in modern France as a medical supplement as well as for maintaining beauty and athletic skill. This type of massage became popular in Japan about 100 years ago when we opened our doors to the West. However, this type of massage does not enter the main stream of medicine in Japan.

Later a modern method of manipulation was imported to Japan that focused on bone structure, the autonomic nervous system, and internal organ functioning rather than on muscle, lymphatic, and blood circulation as is the case with massage. A few traditional anma therapists studied this new method and combined it with their own technique creating his own new method, which was usually named after its originator. All of these techniques were placed under the general name shiatsu. So when we use the term shiatsu we may be speaking about a number of different methods of manipulation.

The Reason and Use of Different Manipulative Therapies

In the *Yellow Emperor's Classic of Internal Medicine*, the Yellow Emperor asked the master of oriental medicine why there are so many methods to treat one constitutional sickness and why each method is effective. The master of oriental medicine replied that environment was the reason for the different methods of treatment. "In the eastern part of this country, the people live near the oceans, eat more fish and protein, and tend to develop skin diseases. In this case, acupuncture is the most effective treatment. The western part of the country is characterized by mountains and desert. The people eat more animal protein and tend to be fat. This in turn causes internal organ malfunctioning which is best remedied with herbal medicine. The northern part of the country is extremely cold so therefore the people have more pastures for dairy farming. The internal organs tend to be cold and develop coughing and mucus problems. So in this case, moxibustion is most effective. The southern part of the country is hot and damp where people generally eat more sour and ripe foods. They are prone to get spasms. Acupuncture is very effective in treating such conditions. In the center of the country which is flat, the people enjoy eating without hard labor. A problem of general weakness is prevalent. So therefore, Do-In and *Ankyo* (anma) are effective." So the saint and genius combined these methods to obtain the most effective total treatment depending on the condition of the patient.

We can understand from this example that the effectiveness of each method depends upon the situation. The layman however may treat someone and succeed in curing the person. Impressed with the success of this treatment, he repeats the same method on another person. If he is lucky enough to treat the same person and condition, he will succeed as previously. Otherwise, he will fail without understanding why.

A professional therapist should ask why he did not succeed and realize that he must not adhere to only one method. Knowledge of a variety of methods will help greatly in determining which method would offer the most effective form of treatment for a particular person and his problem.

Many schools of manipulation insist that their method is more effective than any other. Criticism of one technique in terms of another does not prove that one is more advanced or effective than the other. This attitude, which accounted for the lowering of status of Japanese massage, and failure to recognize more than one method is unfortunate for all; too often it is the patient who ends up suffering. In our eagerness to be objective scientifically, we have become insensitive to the subjective part of any sickness—the patient.

In order to find the most effective treatment for a patient, we should be receptive to many different types of therapy always keeping the patient in mind.

Comparison Between Eastern and Western Medicine

After the Renaissance the rise of natural science did away with superstition and erring knowledge and gave mankind new and correct knowledge. Tremendous progress was made in exploring unknown territories, and a culture was created that was based on natural order. The new concepts developed from the premises of natural science lead more into an enlightened and better world from an ignorant, primitive world. Likewise, in medicine scientists were able to conquer difficult problems and diseases, and began to think they could create a utopia in which there would be no death or disease. In contrast, in eastern medicine there existed a completely opposite idea. For example, *Somon*, a Chinese classic medicine book written 2,000 years ago, says that in ancient time people lived a healthy life past one hundred years of age, but today people are living to only half that age. Is it because the times have changed or is it because people themselves are shortening their lives? This observation is like the Buddhism concept of end-of-the-century decadence, in which man's happy existence progresses to an unhappy one. But before we destroy ourselves completely and disappear, we have some help to bring us back to the ancient way, the better life. Religion and medicine provide that help. This is the concept of oriental decadentism.

In the western idea, mankind started from one dark point and progressed to a bright future. This can be referred to as a direct-line theory. In eastern thought, on the contrary, mankind started from an ideal and saintly world, went to a corrupted and unhappy, disastrous existence, and there regained some of the original, happy state to create a better future.

This is a cyclical theory. In order to understand the order of nature, western so-called straight-line thinking analyzed phenomena and looked for causes, then combined the results and rationalized everything to develop well-systemized theories. But in order to understand and explain the phenomenon of life, western rational thought faced self-contradictions. The latter gave rise to dialectics. Dialectics corresponds to the oriental yin-yang theory, in which a natural phenomenon is understood and explained from a life-cycle point of view.

Straight-line and Cyclical Theories

Let me say a bit more about eastern medicine and western natural science. Medicine developed from man's experience and selected those methods that proved effective. In modern science, we combine to create new reactions, and we manufacture chemically to create modern drugs. Fundamental medical theory evolves from experiments in the tube. The objects of such experimentation are pure cultured germs and infected animals. The theory behind this approach is that if you can delete the germ that started the disease, you can cure the disease. This is the essence of straight-line theory. This concept, in which the infectious germ is rendered harmless, brought about chemical drugs. To look at it one way, in order for bigger life to survive, we have to kill smaller life. Therefore, medical drugs and poison have a paper-thin relationship, for drugs can turn into poison. Chinese herbal medicine consists of plants, animal bones, and minerals. It does not directly attack the disease

Fig. 1   LIFE ON THE EARTH

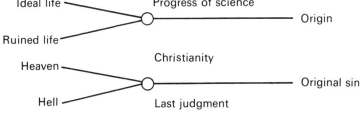

ORIENTAL CYCLICAL THEORY

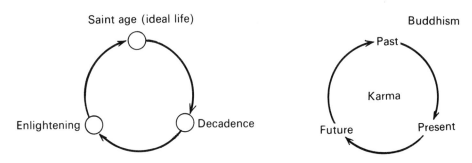

LIFE PHENOMENON

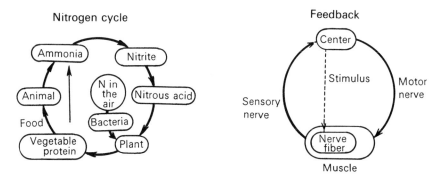

but, instead, helps the living subject that has the disease. Sometimes we make the patient a little worse temporarily in order to cure him completely. The temporarily worsened condition is called *Menken*. In western medicine, doctors control the disease and relieve the pain. In Chinese herbal medicine, according to the condition of the disease, the approach is a circular one in order to cure the disease at its origin. In western medical philosophy, power is used against power on a straight line. In comparison, eastern medicine, with its cyclical theory, takes the condition as it is and works from that point to relieve it.

Likewise, we get life energy through oxygenization which turns sugar into lactic acid and when ATP converts this lactic acid back into sugar. We call this phenomenon the sugar-lactic acid circuit theory, through which a person can be provided eternal energy.

In Buddhism the result from the cause is the cause again. Cause creates result and result creates another cause. This is what we call *karma*. So likewise, our life energy functions in a circle in our bodies.

Folk Medicine

Today we are so accustomed to modern drug therapy that we have forgotten the importance and necessity of realizing our body's own healing powers. Without this force, our bodies would remain in a state of disease. Unfortunately modern science does not recognize any phenomenon that cannot be explained according to scientific logic, so this truth has been ignored by the medical field. This same attitude of the medical profession holds true with regard to folk medicine.

Because its degree of effectiveness cannot be scientifically analyzed or measured, it is considered quackery. However, from an empirical standpoint, there is no doubt that it works and is effective.

There are an increasing number of people who are becoming disillusioned with the side effects of chemical drugs and are turning to folk medicine as an effective alternative. However, overzealousness has lead to articles proclaiming folk remedies as a panacea. This exaggeration is just as detrimental to the public as an article stating that a particular drug can eliminate all diseases because it lacks the basic principle underlying the true meaning of health and sickness. The basic and most important principle underlying health is the balancing of our life force and maintenance and reliance on our body's own natural healing power. Medicine of any kind, be it natural or chemical, are only secondary.

In order for any type of treatment to be effective, it must be understood for what it is—with its limits as well as its potentialities. In order to promote correct knowledge and use of folk medicine, we must view it in proper perspective. The same holds true with shiatsu.

14

The Purpose of Medicine

If we are leading a natural healthy life, there is no need for medicine except in cases of emergency. History has shown us that the state of medicine has often reflected the social condition of the times. During war, a time of social chaos, epidemics were common and the need for medicine prevailed. The classic books stated that the necessity for medicine is an indication that we are living abnormally and not according to nature's laws. In order to cure the disease, we must cure the cause. For example, developing advanced medical techniques to treat wounded soldiers in war mean nothing unless we try to cease having wars. Medicine developed to cure diseases caused by pollution cannot be considered an advancement unless we stop pollution. As long as the medical field concentrates on curing symptoms for diseases caused by our abnormal social and technological disorder, medicine will only contribute toward this abnormal social condition and way of life.

Preventive Medicine

In western medicine, preventive medicine involves early discovery of infections and diseases with immediate treatment; building healthy bodies, and having routine check-ups. But is this really preventive?

General guidelines for preventing diseases from reaching epidemic proportions involve the mass at large, but it does not emphasize the responsiblity an individual should have toward the condition of his own health. Furthermore, in preventive medicine as well as the general medical field, disease is treated as a labeled set of symptoms that apply to everyone.

In oriental medicine, we do not look for a specific disease but instead try to diagnose the unhealthy phenomenon that is occurring in a particular individual. We view the patient in terms of his body as unique from anyone else's and take into consideration his basic constitution. We try to find out why this disease developed in the first place and work from there rather than search for a cure.

In oriental medicine, Dr. Hans Selye's stress theory confirms that we should select the type of treatment according to the phenomenon being observed in the patient rather than following a treatment for a specific disease. In western medicine, there is no way to treat a patient unless a specific disease with specific symptoms is clearly diagnosed. Even preventive medicine works with this basic principle.

Fig. 2

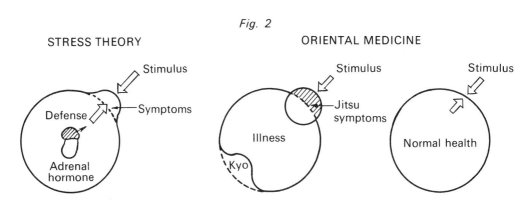

Today there are so many people who are midway between healthy and sick. We may call them "half-healthy" people. We can also call them "next-to-sick" people. There is no positive way for helping them until they become ill in the western sense. In oriental medicine, we can immediately begin treatment to these half-healthy people before naming the disease and even, in fact, while we are waiting for the diagnosis.

In India, they say that ayurvedic medicine is similar to oriental medicine as practiced in Japan; that is, they diagnose the phenomenon occurring in the patient rather than searching for a particular disease. In short, they treat the phenomenon, not the disease.

A very effective treatment can be given if the distortion or abnormal phenomenon is discovered as soon as possible before it develops into a concrete disease that can be categorized. Making an individual aware of his own physical make-up and sensitive to his body when something is not "right" can help greatly in maintaining true health. The whiter the paper, the easier it can show us the dirt; the healthier, the more sensitive one is to distortion. Guiding people to the goal of health with proper care and rest incorporated in our daily lives is preventive medicine in the true sense.

What Shiatsu Does for You

I consider shiatsu to be one of the best health care methods in daily life that can not only treat but prevent disease. Conventional medical treatment is employed only when you have become ill. No medicine can guarantee that you will never be ill with its usage. For instance, vaccination against tuberculosis is not for preventing the infection of tuberculosis but rather for killing the germ before it produces symptoms of the tubercular infection. In addition, this preventive measure is often accompanied by side reactions that can resemble a mild case of the very disease it is trying to prevent. If infection does not occur, the medicine is not only useless, but to some extent, harmful to those with a fundamentally weak constitution. Healthy people will not contract tuberculosis with or without the vaccination.

Chinese herbal medicine, acupuncture, and moxibustion cure symptoms but do not increase physical strength. However, unlike western medicine, they are able to begin early treatment of so-called "half-sick" people, without the side reactions which are often associated with western medicine.

It is important for us to keep in mind that incorporation of shiatsu and a balanced diet into our daily life will keep us healthy. Diet is the root of good health, for it is food that nourishes life. Therefore, proper knowledge of a balanced diet is fundamental to proper health care.

In order for the body to benefit from a balanced diet, it is important that the food is consumed under relaxing conditions that will promote proper digestion. The way we eat and digest our foods is influenced greatly by our social environment. So, to a great extent our health relies on and reflects healthy human relationships.

Basic human relationships are "skin-ships"—that is, skin to skin. In our stress-filled environment, this relationship is constantly being threatened. As a result, a great deal of tension is carried in the skin. This in turn causes cutaneous distortions that eventually affect the functioning of the internal organs.

Shiatsu treatments can give us the opportunity to be aware of not only physical but social distortions. If one is comfortable receiving shiatsu, most likely he has established good human relationships. If he finds it uncomfortable, tension created by his social environment may be a factor in causing internal malfunctioning. In both cases, shiatsu can provide a means of accumulating and establishing better human relationships that are essential for good health.

When we are healthy, our body responds to the external environment in a natural, positive manner. In shiatsu, the giver and receiver create a warm and understanding human relationship through touch and body pressure and become sensitive to each other. Mental and emotional discomfort can be sensed immediately through cutaneous contact. Thus discomfort and abnormal functioning of the mind and body can be transmitted between practitioner and patient through shiatsu. In some instances this discomfort is not felt until a later time. Discomfort produced by external stimulation in the form of pressure can make us aware of our natural self-healing power. By sensing his distortion, the patient is given an opportunity to become aware of it and consider its cause. If his condition is not serious, he can depend on his own physical resources to get well. People lacking in self-awareness can benefit from shiatsu by having the discomfort which he feels tune into what is happening to his body. By making the patient aware of these phenomena, the shiatsu practitioner can guide the patient back to a normal life.

It is the job of the practitioner to be sincere in sharing his knowledge with his patients. He should not be critical of a patient's weakness, but instead be compassionate toward his patient's pain.

2. Zen Shiatsu and Its Theory

Definition of Shiatsu

The Japanese Ministry of Health and Welfare states "Shiatsu therapy is a form of manipulation administered by the thumbs, fingers, and palms, without the use of any instrument, mechanical or otherwise, to apply pressure to the human skin, correct internal malfunctioning, promote and maintain health, and treat specific diseases."

Ancient Japanese massage (anma), modern massage, and shiatsu can be categorized according to the manner in which manual stimulation is given. Shiatsu can also be defined as the application of "one-point" pressure that combines many varieties of rhythmical and changing stimulation. All three methods of manipulation aim at stabilizing the functioning of the human body, the difference being in whether they stimulate blood circulation and nerve erections directly or indirectly. The effectiveness of manipulative therapy has been proven by modern scientific experiments involving cutaneous stimulation. From this point of view, no difference exists among the basic three techniques, though they were developed from different principles.

The three techniques are legally classified as different, but professionals themselves admit that there is little reason to do so. The purpose of manipulative therapy is to heal people by working with a person's natural healing force to correct any internal malfunctioning peculiar to that person. The name shiatsu was employed to distinguish it as a form of treatment rather than something given only for pleasure.

Shiatsu as a Medical Treatment

As mentioned previously, geographical environment greatly influences the type of disease and medicine used in a particular location. Medical technique must be chosen by the condition of the patient. Western medicine developed in order to treat diseases like the plague of the Middle Ages or cancer in modern times, and developed for emergency medicine. Oriental medicine developed according to the oriental geography and natural environment, so when it came to Japan, it had to be converted for the Japanese environment. Differences in Japanese massage (anma), European massage, and shiatsu lie in the social demands from which they developed. Anma and European massage directly stimulate blood circulation emphasizing the release of stagnated blood in the skin and muscles and tension and stiffness resulting from circulatory congestion. On the other hand, shiatsu emphasizes correction and maintenance of bone structure, joints, tendons, muscles, and meridian lines whose malfunctioning distort the body's energy and autonomic nervous system causing disease.

Shiatsu as a home remedy is also effective though accurate diagnosis is necessary for positive professional results. A while ago, I published a book titled *Shiatsu in Your Home* in Japanese. The main purpose of this book was to shed a new light on shiatsu for the professional practitioner.

However, I was surprised to receive so many letters from laymen reporting tremendous results with their family and friends. The technique and theory behind it were fully understood and practiced by them.

It is impossible for the layman to practice acupuncture, chiropractic, and osteopathy; even trained professionals need time and understanding to master these techniques. On the other hand, shiatsu is simple, effective, and safe. These are the elements of its popularity as home medicine. One hundred fifty years ago, Shinsai Ota wrote a book on *Ampuku* shiatsu emphasizing that honest, sincere, and simple shiatsu is much better than merely technique-oriented professional shiatsu.

Shiatsu Diagnosis

The line between amateur and professional shiatsu does not lie in the number of techniques one can use; rather the professional should have a more thorough understanding of the tsubo theory and how it works and is applied. Ironically enough, the more shiatsu is exaggerated as being easy, the more people turn to professional shiatsu for help.

Shiatsu on a professional level requires accurate diagnosing in order to determine what is the best treatment for a particular patient. Without correct diagnostic skill, the shiatsu therapist cannot go beyond mere "home remedy" treatments. In shiatsu, treatment is diagnosis, diagnosis is treatment. In oriental medicine, four methods of observing phenomena are used: *bo-shin*; general diagnosis through observation; *bun-shin*; diagnosis through sound; *mon-shin*; diagnosis through questioning; and *setsu-shin*; diagnosis through touch. In shiatsu, *setsu-shin* or diagnosis through touch is the final method that determines the condition of the patient. In *setsu-shin* or touching diagnosis, the body must be considered as a whole, so the techniques used in this type of diagnosis are for discovering malfunctionings of the total body.

One technique used in oriental medicine as part of *setsu-shin* is the pulse technique. In western medicine the pulse indicates heart palpitations, but in oriental medicine it is used to diagnose the condition of the twelve meridians. You can feel what meridian lines are *kyo* and *jitsu* in the pulse area.

Another technique is ampuku therapy or *setsu-shin* on the *hara* area. The master of oriental medicine, Toudou Yoshimasu once said, "*Hara* is the source of *Ki* energy. All disease stems from this area. Therefore, you can feel everything by diagnosing the hara." This is the basic principle underlying hara diagnosis in Japanese massage. In ampuku therapy, there is no need to rub down or massage the hara area—simply apply steady and continuous pressure.

Pressure should be held from three to seven seconds for effective results. If you press quickly, you will not give deep stimulation. By applying steady or continuous pressure on the skin, pain will gradually subside and you will be able to feel more clearly the true condition of that area of the body. The more concentrated the area of pressure, the more effective response you will receive.

Shiatsu also deals with the sympathetic and parasympathetic nervous system. Both systems work together in regulating the body and its activities. For example, when you suddenly hear an unexpected noise there is an immediate reaction from the sympathetic nervous system. When the noise dies down, the parasympathetic nervous system becomes active by making the person feel sleepy.

The same holds true on the skin. Sharp changes cause stimulation of the sympathetic nervous system increasing heart palpitations. This is the purpose of western massage. In order to affect the functioning of the internal organs, however, the parasympathetic nervous system must be stimulated. In short, to stimulate the body, the sympathetic nerves come into play; to sedate the parasympathetic nerves become active.

By applying continuous steady pressure, we can control the reaction of the sympathetic nerves and work with the parasympathetic nervous system. The method for reaching the parasympathetic nerves involves the use of both hands simultaneously. By using the palm of one hand and the fingertips of the other, you will be able to feel in the palm the changes that take place while you press with the fingertips of your other hand. When the parasympathetic nervous system reacts negatively, you will feel resistance against the pressure you are exerting. This resistance should not be taken for tightness in a particular area, but rather understood as a reaction from the autonomic nervous system. Thus any discomfort created by the incorrect quality and quantity of pressure is felt mutually by practitioner and patient.

Sympathy and compassion for the patient is very important in oriental diagnosis. Unfortunately, western medical techniques ignore a patient's condition if it does not comply with their standards of sickness or disease, often labeling it as a condition of anxiety and leaving it at that. Touching diagnosis is maternal affection toward the patient to feel his pain. This means that we are not treating the patient's problem but rather sharing his pain. It is important that we remember this when giving shiatsu in order to avoid reducing the treatment to superficial fingertip technique. As long as *setsu-shin* is emphasized and practiced, shiatsu will not be reduced to a massage merely for pleasure.

Manipulation and Touching Diagnosis

The classic Chinese medicine books state that *kyo* and *jitsu* must first be found in the meridian lines by touching or kneading before administering acupuncture or moxibustion. After the treatment is completed, the same initial procedure of touching is repeated. Even though you stimulate the meridian lines with acupuncture or moxibustion, better results can be achieved with the addition of touching diagnosis. Modern acupuncture techniques, however, do not use *setsu-shin* and therefore need to insert more needles to achieve the desired results.

Though the four methods of diagnosis which I mentioned already seem difficult, in actuality all it requires is that the patient be observed as a rule carefully. His breathing pattern, irregular reactions such as coughing, and conduct should be instinctively understood by the practitioner. Western physicians believe that drugs and operations can cure disease and regard the diagnostic method as simply routine greetings. They fail to realize the important role these "greetings" play in making the patient feel familiar and secure with the doctor. Real medicine begins the moment the doctor places his hands on the patient's hara. Drugs and operations are the last resort. In shiatsu, this kind of touching is already treatment.

Touching diagnosis is not only an instinctive form of manipulation but also a concrete expression of a human relationship that can greatly affect the results of any medical treatment. In shiatsu this "skin-ship" relationship is created by dealing with the discomfort directly using touching diagnosis.

Oriental *setsu-shin* requires that the practitioner apply steady and firm pressure that relaxes the sympathetic nervous system and allows the parasympathetic nervous system to calm the functioning of the internal organs. Unlike western touching diagnosis in which the doctor looks for the condition of the skin, muscle, and internal organ by stimulating the sympathetic nervous system resulting in a strong reaction, oriental touching diagnosis *setsu-shin* is performed with instinctive compassion and without scare. The patient is better able to let the practitioner feel the real condition of his body. In many cases the practitioner is able to feel more than the patient the general condition of his body.

According to the philosophy of yin and yang, yin is silent and motionless, while yang is surface and active. The combination of the two must be taken into consideration when treating diseases. The symptoms that appear on the surface are yang while the root of the disease which is deep and hidden is yin. Without understanding the root of the disease, which is difficult to find, the disease will not be cured. To illustrate my point, take for instance grass. Grass grows above the earth and is yang, the roots below, yin. It is easy to find the part that grows above the earth but difficult to find the part below. No matter how many times you cut the grass, it grows back sooner or later unless you pull out the roots. The same applies to shiatsu. You cannot cure disease by treating only the yang part.

Shiatsu and Meridian Lines

In western medicine the concept of meridian lines has not been proven scientifically. However, just like Chinese herbal medicine which is not manufactured in a scientific laboratory, it is sometimes more effective than conventional scientific drugs. Some acupuncture methods only deal with the tsubos or in English acu-points, ignoring the meridian lines theory, but I cannot deny the very effectiveness of treating tsubos relates to meridian lines.

Meridian lines are defined as channels of living magnetic energy in the body. Sometimes these channels can be associated with the functioning of the internal organs. Long before modern medicine acknowledged the relationship that exists between the skin and internal organs. The Orient developed a system of treating disease by stimulating points on the skin that were connected to the functioning of the internal organs. These points were connected by an imaginary line to form meridian lines and were used mainly in acupuncture and moxibustion.

Then Drs. Yoshio Nagahama and Masao Maruyama published a report citing that signs of a specific disease appeared on the surface of the patient's body like small indentations beneath the skin. The pattern of these indentations were very similar to conventional acupuncture meridian lines.

Meridian lines and systemized tsubos are believed to have come into existence through acupuncture, but I believe that manual manipulation was the first to use them. As I mentioned in another section of this book, the classic acupuncture treatment began and ended with *setsu-shin* or touching diagnosis which revealed an accurate diagnosis of the body's condition.

Through my own experience, I have found that you can feel the meridian lines by pressing on the correct tsubos, even though you may not be a supersensitive practitioner. I have also discovered that the tsubos connect with other tsubos forming wider meridian lines that are not straight. These meridian lines, I have found, cover the whole body and are more numerous than the conventional acupuncture meridian lines.

Recently other therapies such as auricular therapy, foot reflexology, and iridology have been used as diagnostic measures for determining the condition of the entire body. Taking these theories into consideration, acknowledging only six meridians in the arms, six in the legs and more or less 600 tsubos on the entire body is a rather simplified way of viewing the body. Dr. Nagahama has reported that he has found two or three additional meridian lines. Judging from my clinical experience, I find twelve meridian lines in the arms and legs that pass through the back, hara, neck, and head.

In classical oriental medicine there are fourteen major meridian lines. In manipulation we should not be limited by the meridian lines as is the case with acupuncture. We can add on to the conventional meridian lines, because in manipulation we deal with a wider area. In my treatments so far I have found twelve meridians in the legs and twelve meridians in arms. Treating these meridians have produced more effective results.

22

Fig. 3

━ ━ ━ Lung Meridian   ━━━━━ Large Intestine Meridian

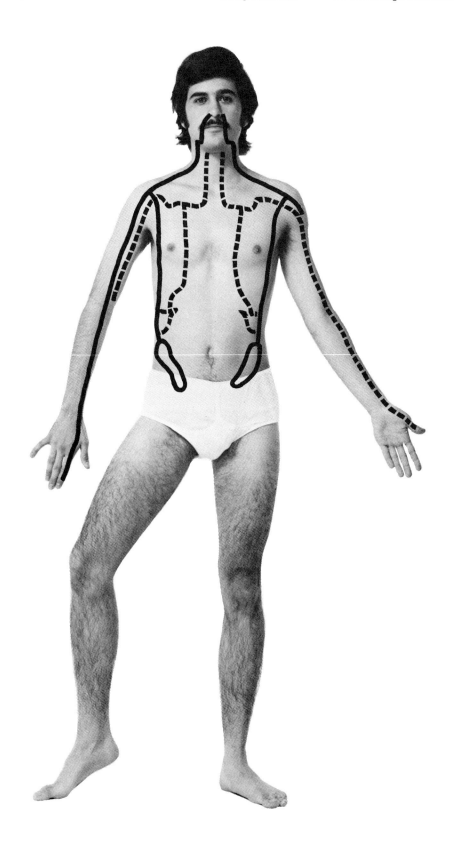

Fig. 4

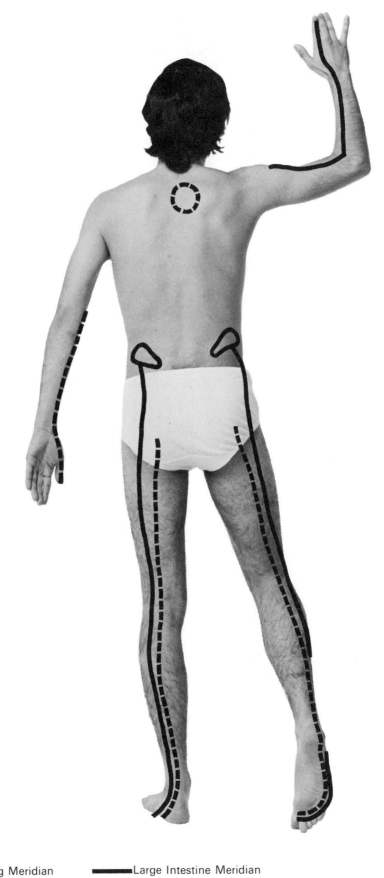

▬ ▬ ▬Lung Meridian　　　▬▬▬▬Large Intestine Meridian

24

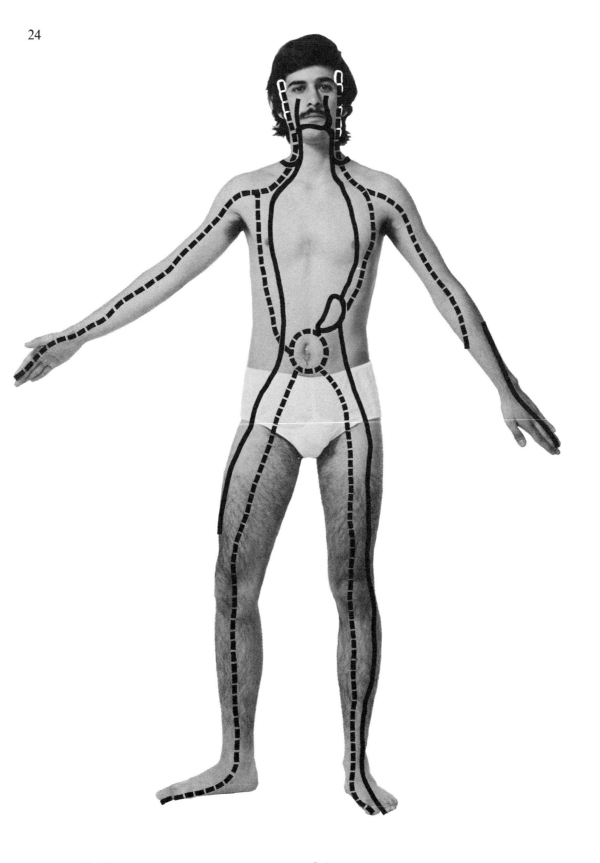

Fig. 5   ■■■■Spleen Meridian   ■■■■■■Stomach Meridian

Fig. 6

■ ■ ■ ■Spleen Meridian
━━━Stomach Meridian

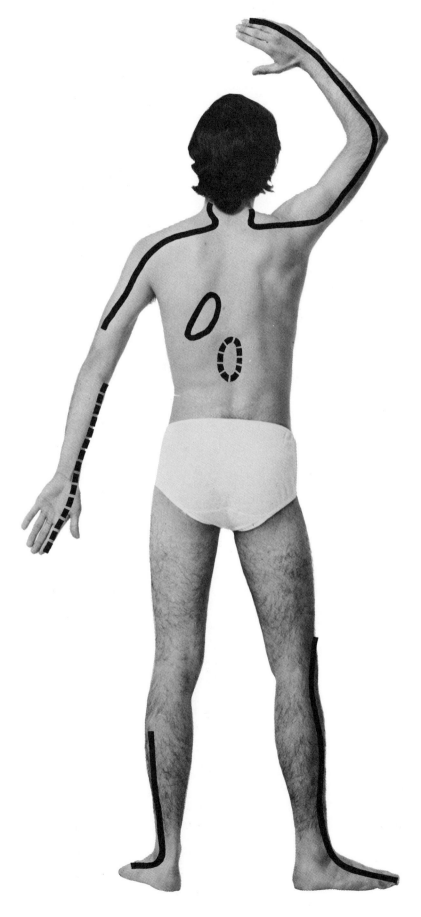

Fig. 7

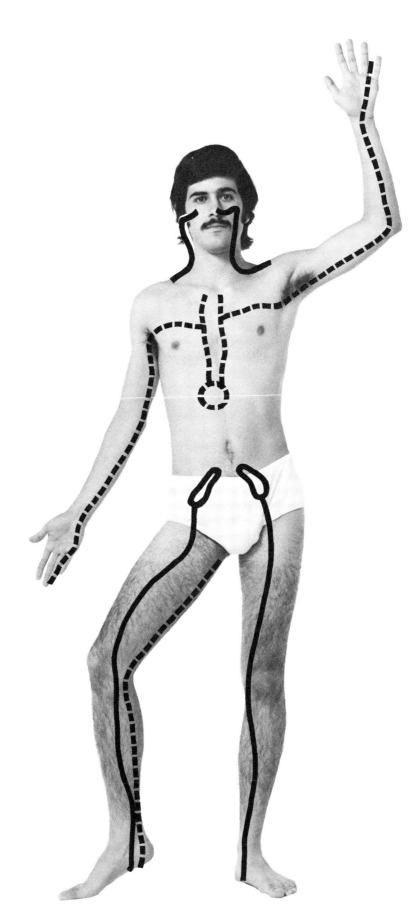

▬ ▬ ▬Heart Meridian
▬▬▬Small Intestine
Meridian

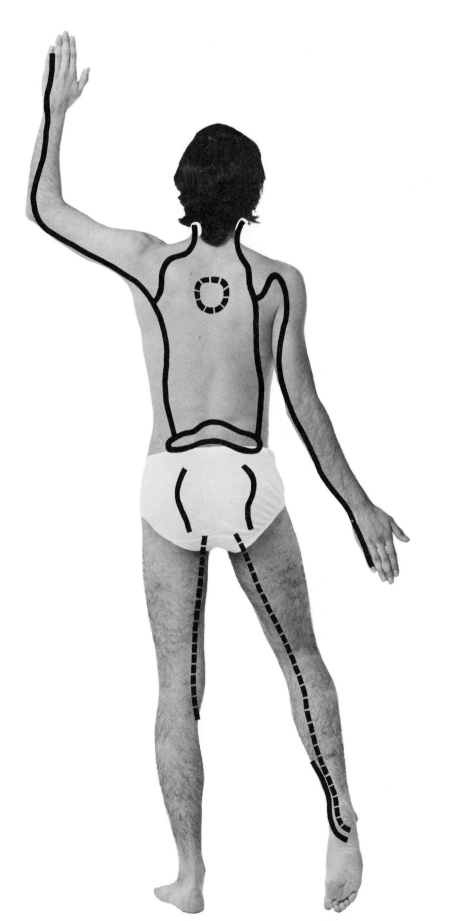

Fig. 8

∎ ∎ ∎ ∎Heart Meridian

▬▬▬▬Small Intestine
Meridian

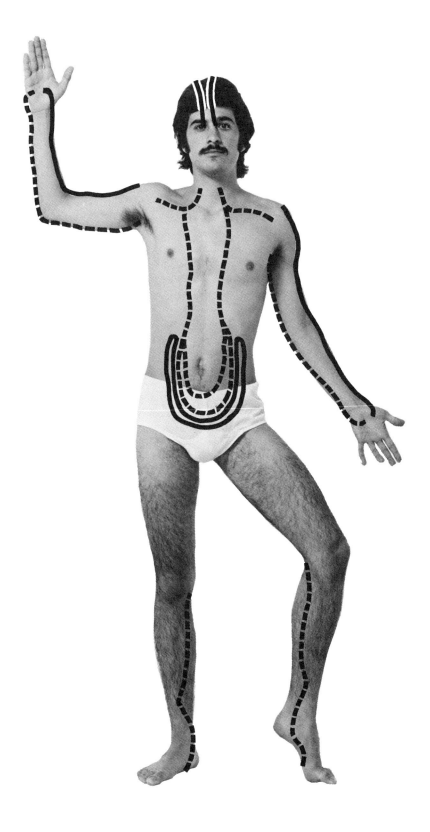

Fig. 9   ▪▬ ▬▪Kidney Meridian   ▬▬▬▬Bladder Meridian

Fig. 10 ▬▬■■Kidney Meridian ▬▬▬Bladder Meridian

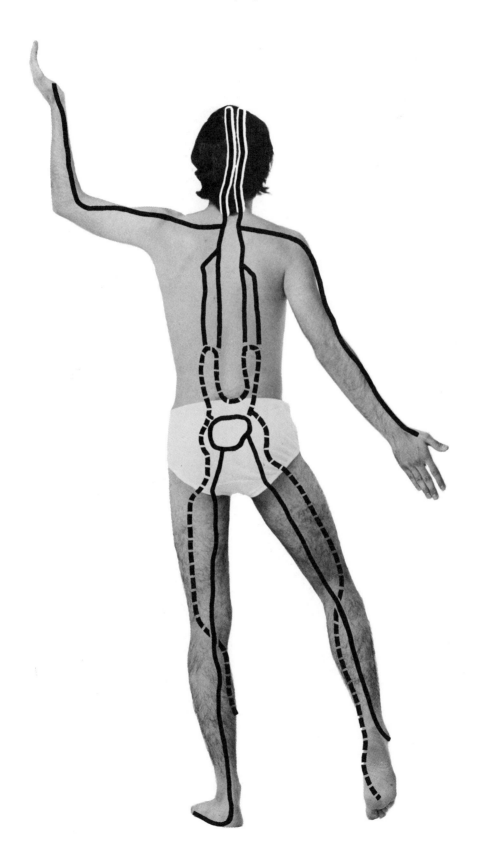

Fig. 11 ▬ ▬ ▬▬Heart Constrictor Meridian   ▬▬▬▬Triple Heater Meridian

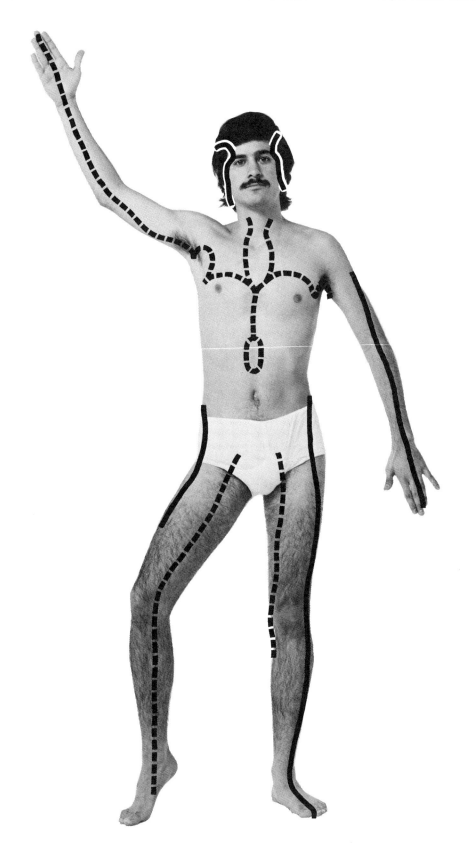

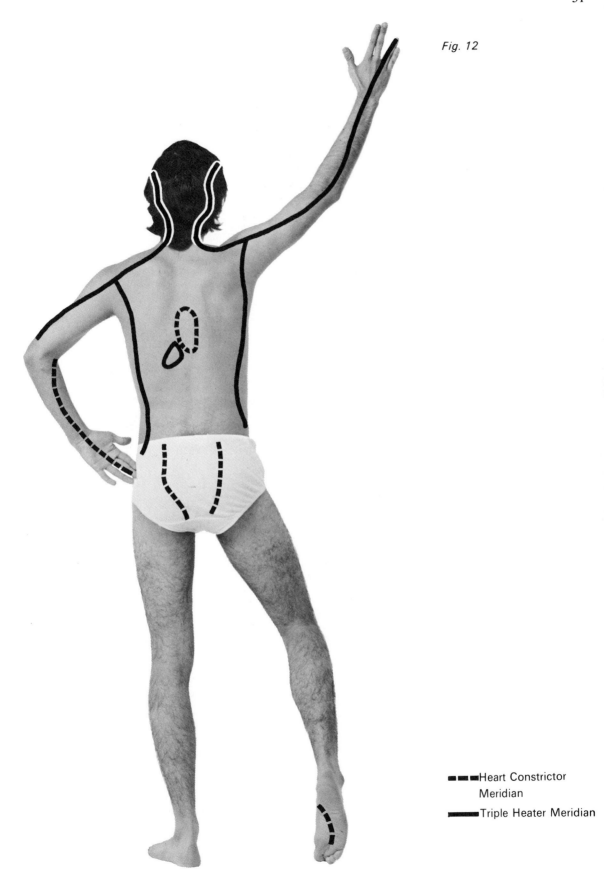

Fig. 12

■■■Heart Constrictor
Meridian

■■■Triple Heater Meridian

32

Fig. 13

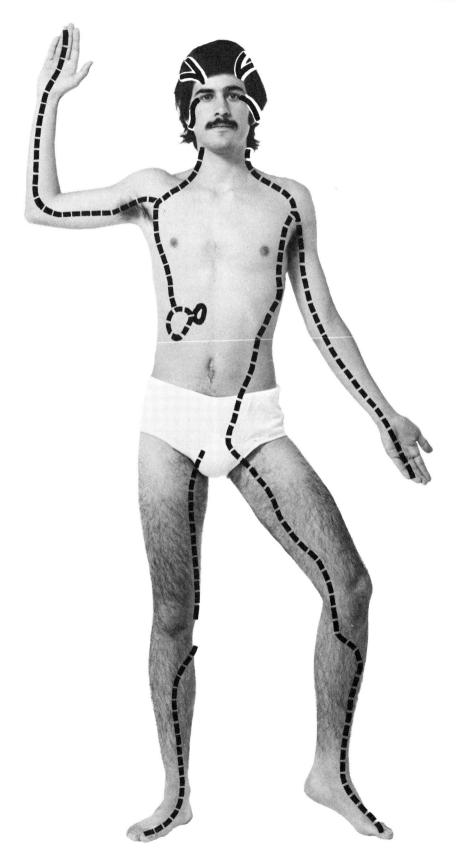

Fig. 14

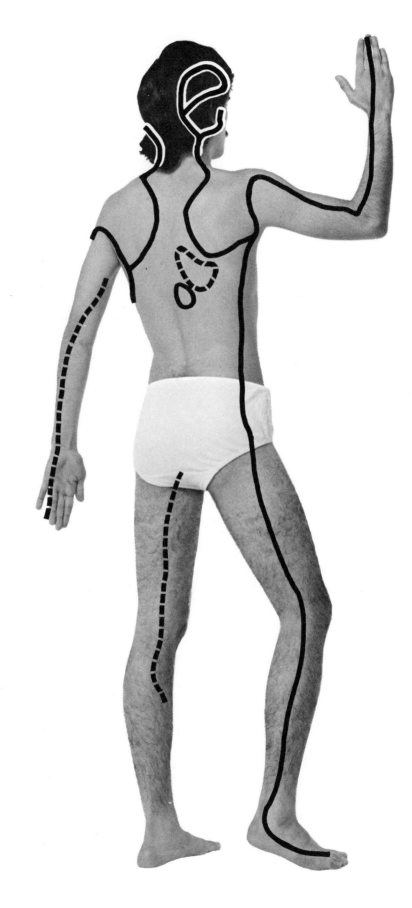

▬ ▬ ▬Liver Meridian

▬▬▬Gall Bladder
Meridian

Fig. 15   ▄▄▄▄Yin Meridian   ▄▄▄▄Yang Meridian

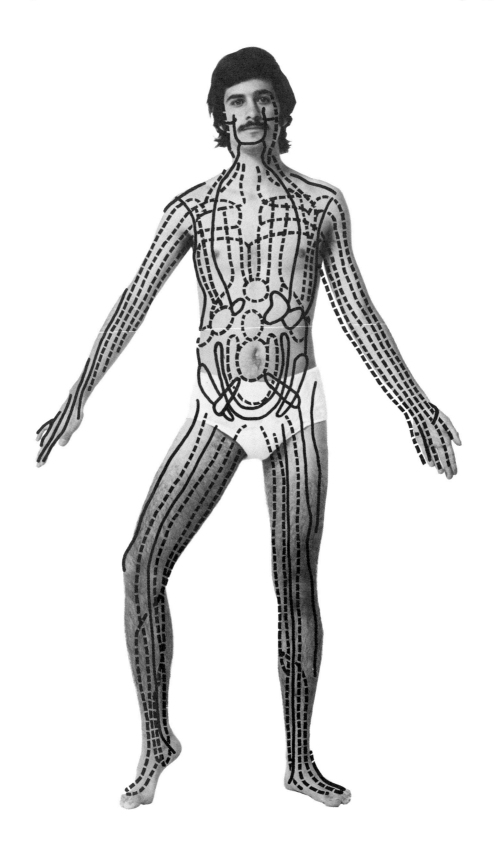

Fig. 16

━━━Yin Meridian ━━━━Yang Meridian

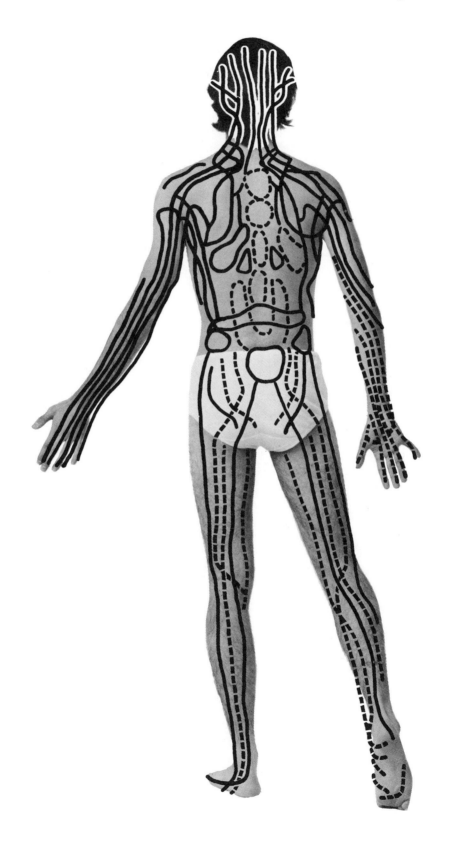

36

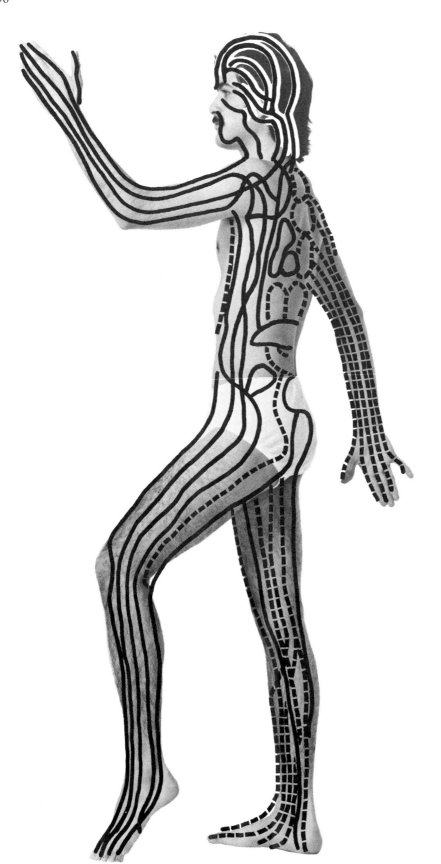

Fig. 17

====Yin Meridian
===Yang Meridian

Using this system of meridian lines I developed a manipulative technique that can be used instead of the pulse to diagnose accurately along the arms and legs.

To do this meridian stretching technique, hold the pivot point firmly with one hand and stretch the appendage in the direction of the arrow as seen in Fig. 18. By doing this, the meridian lines will surface on the skin enabling you to diagnose clearly whether the meridian is *kyo* or *jitsu*.

You find by using this technique that the *jitsu* condition will appear as hard but elastic in a state of resistance, and sometimes actually protruding from the meridian. The *kyo* area will feel flabby even in the maximum stretch position. The area will seem weak with stiffness found after deep penetration. This technique is more effective than ordinary *setsu-shin*.

Fig. 18

STRETCHING MERIDIANS

ARMS

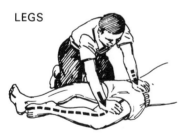

LU (lung meridian) greater yin (LI—large intestine meridian)

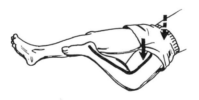

HC (heart constrictor meridian) absolute yin (TH—triple heater meridian)

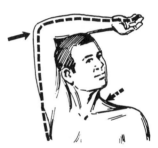

HT (heart meridian) lesser yin (SI—small intestine meridian)

LEGS

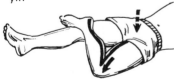

SP (spleen meridian) greater yin

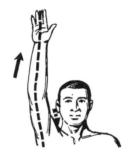

SI greater yang

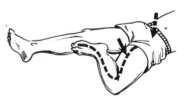

LV (liver meridian) absolute yin

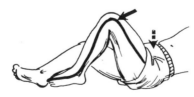

BL (bladder meridian) greater yang

TH lesser yang

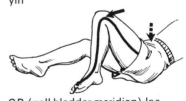

GB (gall bladder meridian) lesser yang

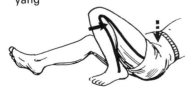

LI sunlight yang

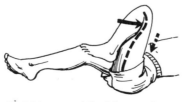

KI (kidney meridian) lesser yin

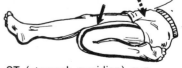

ST (stomach meridian) sunlight yang

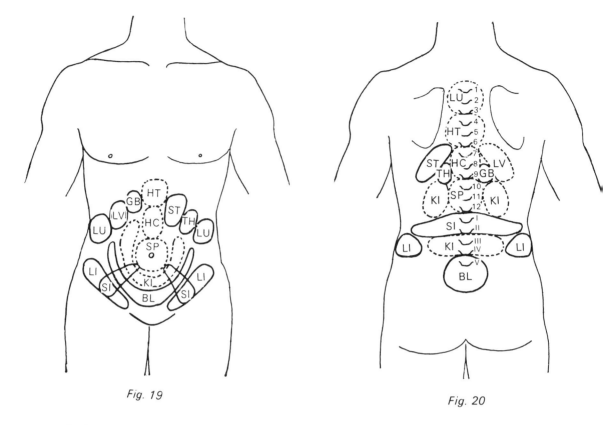

Fig. 19   Fig. 20

In hara and back diagnosis (Figs. 19 and 20) you can feel what meridians are *kyo* and *jitsu* by feeling the area related to each of the twelve meridians. After diagnosing *kyo* and *jitsu* you can give shiatsu using the tonification-sedation technique.

The Importance of Kyo and Jitsu on the Meridians

The energy that maintains our vital life force flows through twelve pathways called meridians. The quality of energy perceived in these meridians can be divided into three yang qualities; sunlight yang, greater yang, and lesser yang; and three yin qualities; absolute yin, greater yin, and lesser yin. The posterior part of the body is yang while the anterior part is yin. Therefore, the arm and leg both have three yin and three yang meridians with a total of twelve meridians passing through the limbs.

In addition to the twelve "regular" meridians there are eight additional ones which come into play in cases of emergency. The governing vessel which is yang, and the conception vessel which is yin are exceptional meridians because they run down the center of the body. The twelve meridians are named after six "Zo" and six "Fu" organs. However, the relation between the organ and meridian exists in the functioning of the organ rather than the organ itself.

Under healthy conditions, the energy flows freely through these meridians in a balanced state. When abnormal functioning of the internal organs or abnormal external stimulation occurs, energy stagnates in the meridians producing sickness.

Therefore, in order to cure the disease, the energy must be released and normalized.

In order to do this first diagnose where the stagnation is and then stimulate the meridian involved. You can work on the entire meridian evenly or concentrate on specific points on the meridian. In either case, the flow of energy will be normalized.

When stagnation is not serious and easily released, this indicates that strength still remains in the patient's energy system and he is more the *jitsu* type. If his energy is depleted to such an extent that chronic stagnation occurs, he is more the *kyo* type. *Kyo* type people are more difficult to cure because overstimulation can worsen the condition. In these cases, accurate diagnosis is essential in treating *kyo* type people.

Kyo and Jitsu—Tonification and Sedation

The condition of energy (called *Ki* in Japanese) in the meridian lines is defined by *kyo* and *jitsu*. These concepts are very similar to yin and yang. *Kyo* is the condition of depleted energy, which is more hypo, while *jitsu* is the condition of excess energy, which is more hyper. We can illustrate this by thinking of a perfectly round ball representing a healthy person. Now think of a distorted ball with indentations and protrusions marring its circumference (Fig. 21). The indentations which are hollow and below the surface are the areas of *kyo*. The protrusions are *jitsu*. Obviously it is much easier to spot the *jitsu* areas because they project from the surface, but it is much more difficult to find the *kyo* areas which are the cause of the problem. This concept of *kyo* and *jitsu* is known in classic Chinese medical books as *jya-ki* or the condition of energy distortion. It is important to remember that this condition of distortion is relative to the healing power and constitution of each individual. How a person manifests his sickness in terms of *kyo* or *jitsu* determines the ability of the body to normalize itself.

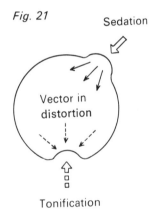

Fig. 21

Sedation

Vector in distortion

Tonification

The technique used to normalize *jitsu* points is called sedation; to normalize *kyo* areas, tonification. In sedation, the *jitsu* area is simply stimulated and the protrusion will normalize itself. However, the hollow areas of *kyo* require patiently holding shiatsu. This takes more time because warmth must reach deep inside to nurture strength to normalize the area. The classic medical books compare tonification with a lover waiting for his love's arrival—affectionately, patiently, and without regard to time.

It is easier to find the *jitsu* areas and sedate them than it is to find the *kyo* areas and strengthen them. If a person maintains a strong healing power in his body, *jitsu* areas can be normalized with simple sedation without much difficulty. The chronic *kyo* patient on the other hand has more difficulty in normalizing his energy because his body's healing power has been depleted due to extreme fatigue. In this case correct tonification techniques should be used. If you stimulate the *jitsu* areas of a chronically *kyo* patient negligently, you may cause the patient to consume what energy he has and thus worsen the condition. Unnecessary sedation to chronically *kyo* patients can cause further imbalance, so be sure that you find the *kyo* areas before proceeding with treatment.

It is sometimes tempting to try to prove yourself by working on the obviously *jitsu* areas, but as an old oriental proverb states, "behind every crime, there is a woman," so behind every yang or *jitsu* condition there is a yin or *kyo* condition. Because *kyo* is fundamental to any disease, it must be tonified in order to cure the disease.

According to western medicine's straight line theory, you simply attack the symptoms and cure them without regard to the body as a whole. In oriental medicine, the round cyclical theory approaches the problem by trying to improve the patient's constitution. Chinese herbal medicine, acupuncture, and moxibustion are similar to western medicine in that the techniques involved are for sedation. In Chinese herbal medicine as well as homeopathy, poison is given to kill the poison causing the problem. In the cases of acupuncture and moxibustion, you kill the pain by giving pain. On the other hand, diet and manipulation are more moderate and self-healing and less harmful though difficult to understand. Even if your diagnosis is incorrect, strong reactions cannot occur through improper treatment, Accurate diagnosis, *kyo* and *jitsu*, and proper tonification-sedation techniques are especially important for the professional.

Meridian Diagnosis

In shiatsu, meridian diagnosis is the best way to understand the condition of a patient's disease. Unlike chiropractic and osteopathy which concentrate on distortions of the bone structure, we deal with total functional distortions in terms of the meridian lines.

Meridian diagnosis requires that you feel *kyo* and *jitsu* on two meridian lines. Then you give tonification to one meridian and sedation to the other. Other forms of therapy such as acupuncture are basically more sedative, so manipulation can complement this by giving tonification.

We usually do not generalize about *kyo* and *jitsu* in relation to the *zo-fu* organs from the theory of the five elements. For instance, we do not think of bladder meridian only as *jitsu* and kidney meridian as *kyo*. Instead we have found that if one meridian in one element is *kyo*, its corresponding meridian in the same element will also have the same condition in comparison with the other four elements and their meridians. For example, if we find the lung meridian *kyo*, most likely the large intestine will also be *kyo* in comparison to the other meridians.

Classic Chinese medical books state that every *kyo* has *jitsu* in it and vice versa. If you compare two meridian lines within one element (for example, lung and large intestine meridians) one meridian will be more *kyo* or *jitsu* than the other. If you can diagnose and feel the *kyo* within *kyo* (meaning *kyo* as compared with the other meridians of the four elements) and *jitsu* within *jitsu* (the condition *jitsu* as compared with the other meridians of the four elements) then you can treat the most *kyo* and most *jitsu* areas. Of course, you do not have to limit this method to only two meridians in order to find *kyo* and *jitsu*. The condition of *kyo* and *jitsu* appears more or less on all the meridian lines because disease affects the total body.

The best method is to choose the most *kyo* and most *jitsu* meridian lines and concentrate on tonifying and sedating them. Lesser degrees of distortion can be eliminated by recovery of the areas of the biggest distortion. If good results are not achieved through tonification, an inaccurate diagnosis is at fault and should be checked. There are 120 possible combinations of *kyo* and *jitsu* in the twelve meridian lines when each meridian is coupled with a meridian under the same element. The Japanese say that there are 404 types of disease, within which 10,000 diseased conditions appear. All occur within the 120 phenomena described above. Because phenomena change from day to day, the diagnosis made cannot indicate the seriousness of the disease nor pinpoint what category of disease or distortion has caused the condition being observed. This constantly changing distortion is influenced greatly by the healing power within the body. Therefore simply tonify or sedate the affected meridians according to the diagnosis made at the time of treatment. Sometimes you may find a phenomenon constitutionally very deep and at other times very acute. Small distortions may disappear during the treatment and can be confirmed through hara diagnosis. Toudou, the master of oriental medicine, once said that the hara always comes first. If you apply this theory to shiatsu you can diagnose the total body condition and treat it effectively through tonification and sedation techniques. When you are diagnosing you are actually giving a life diagnosis. That means that you are not looking for a specific disease but improving the patient's life by working from the roots of his existence and enlightening the patient to a better way of life.

Fig. 22

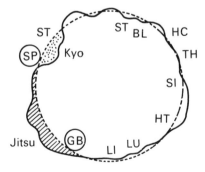

SP kyo

GB jitsu

Lung and Large Intestine Meridians—Analysis of Function of Elimination

Function of the Lung Meridian		Intake of *Ki* energy which is fundamental in life from the air for use by the human body and to build up resistance against external intrusions. Elimination of gases not needed through the process of exhalation.	
		Psychological	Physical
Lung Meridian	*Kyo*	Mental collapse, strong palpitations, hypersensitivity, overanxiety, breathing difficulties, antisocial, short breath.	Prone to be overweight with elimination difficulties. Heaviness in the head because of blood stagnation. Upper part of body prone to fatigue and coughing, difficulty in breathing and lying in prone position, easily susceptible to cold, inflammation in the respiratory organs. Shoulder pain with slight fever, tendency to easily tear and cough. Lack of *Ki* energy and fatigue from overwork, lack of circulation and fatigue in the thumb.
	Jitsu	Obsessed with anxiety over small details with inability for release. Tendency to sigh and choke while breathing.	Prone to nasal congestion, colds. Coughing pain in chest, constipation, shoulder pain, bronchitis, asthma, and mucus. Thumb senses a pulling pain, chest muscles are tight.
Function of the Large Intestine Meridian		Helps the function of the lung. Secretes and excretes from inside and outside of the body. Eliminates the stagnation of *Ki* energy.	
		Psychological	Physical
Large Intestine Meridian	*Kyo*	Lack of determination, tendency to be disappointed, over-dependency, lack of positive thinking. *co-dependency*	Dry or congested nasal passage; weak bronchial tubes, constipation; prone to diarrhea when digesting coarse foods; poor circulation in the lower area of the hara; tendency to shiver. Malfunctioning of the large intestine; no strength in the thumb and lower part of the body below the hips. Lack of vitality in facial expression; easily susceptible to inflammation and pus.
	Jitsu	Perpetual dissatisfaction; no friend with whom he can confer.	Headaches causing a flushed complexion; running nose; nasal congestion, nose bleeding; prone to tonsillitis, painful sensation in the lower teeth; whitish eyes, shoulder pain; stiffness in the chest and arm muscles (located on the thumb side); constipation but occasional diarrhea. Tendency to overeat; headaches; itchy skin, prone to inflammations, lack of exercise, coughing, puffiness in lower hara and hemorrhoids; epilepsy; tendency to catch cold.

Spleen and Stomach Meridians—Function of Digestion and Zymosis

Function of the Spleen Meridian		Digestion and process of fermentation. Spleen is considered to be the pancreas in modern terms and governs general digestion including saliva, gastric bile; secretions from the small intestine; reproductive hormones related to the breast and ovaries. Mental fatigue adversely affects the spleen and lack of exercise causes malfunctioning digestion and hormone secretion.	
		Psychological	Physical
Spleen Meridian	Kyo	Overconcern for details; restless with anxiety; always dissatisfied; tendency to overeat and eat quickly; overuse of the brain; loss of memory; sleepiness.	Lack of gastric acid causing anemia; lack of saliva; sticky and dry taste in the mouth, thirsty; unable to consume food without liquid; inability to taste food; continual eating; brownish color in the face, lack of exercise resulting in poor circulation in the legs and feet; poor digestion; stiff sensation deep in the navel; frequently breathing the air; pale color in gums, pain in the spine.
	Jitsu	Tendency not to talk to others and remain alone; hesitant and timid; tendency to think too much. Cautious and anxious; eats quickly or out of obligation in spite of no exercise; mental unrest, craving for sweets.	Thirsty, sticky feeling in mouth, no appetite, no appreciation for tasting foods, gastric hyperacidity, nervous stomach inflammations, overeating, obesity, heaviness in the legs, no strength, stiffness in the arms, tight feeling in navel area, shallow skin, hesitancy in movement, stiff shoulders, tendency to round back, coldness in the back and the hip area.
Function of the Stomach Meridian		Related to functioning of stomach, esophagus, duodenum, as well as functioning of reproductive, lactation, ovary, and appetite mechanism. Also related to menstrual cycle.	
		Psychological	Physical
Stomach Meridian	Kyo	Tendency to recline and rest, craving for cold and soft food, appetite influenced by mood and quality of food, consumption of food without thorough mastication, tendency to eat while doing something, irregular meals, thinking too much.	Bad stomach, chronic gastric problem, hanging stomach, eating with no appetite, coldness in stomach and intestines; shoulder pain due to ovary problems, yawning, fat legs, easily fatigues; tendency to develop empyemas; coldness felt in the front part of body; lack of flexibility in the muscles.
	Jitsu	Tendency to think too much; nervous about details; frustrated, lacking in affection; big eater, always in a hurry, over working; neurotic.	Overeating; heaviness in the stomach, vomiting, gastric hyperacidity, cold sores, poor appetite, thirsty, stiffness in the shoulder, pain and stiffness in the solar plexus and the heart. Symptoms of catching a cold or the flu, poor circulation in the leg; rough skin, dry complexion, belching and yawning, nasal stagnation, redness on top of the nose, tendency to be anemic, malfunctioning of female organs.

Heart and Small Intestine Meridians—Adaptation and Governing Function

Function of the Heart Meridian		Represents compassion and therefore governs emotions and spirits as well as blood circulation and total body via the brain and five senses. Also functions as the mechanism that adapts external stimuli to the body's internal envirionment	
		Psychological	Physical
Heart Meridian	Kyo	Mental fatigue, shock, nervous tension, stress, neurosis, oversensitivity, poor appetite, restless, lack of memory, anxious, timid, tendency to be disappointed, no will power.	Lack of strength in upper part of hara, tightness in the solar plexus area, strong palpitations, heart organ problems, tension in the hara. Pulling sensation in the tongue, sweaty palms, easily fatigued, pectoral angina condition, coated tongue, myocardiac infraction.
	Jitsu	Chronic tension and stiffness in chest; tries to contain anxiety and restlessness, perpetual fatigue, tendency to stammer, stiffness in the solar plexus area, thirsty, obsession with tonsillitic cancer, laughing.	Pulling sensation in tongue, always clearing the throat, protrusion in the solar plexus and tightness in the heart area, stiff body, hysteria, sweaty palms, easily perspires, sensitive skin, shoulder pain, fever in the stomach area, desire for cold drinks, cardiac nervousness, nervous stomach, palpitation.
Function of the Small Intestine Meridian		Through displacement and digestion of food, small intestine governs total body. Mental anxiety, emotional excitement, nervous shock and anger can affect blood circulation and small intestine causes blood stagnation which affects the entire body.	
		Psychological	Physical
Small Intestine Meridian	Kyo	Tendency to think too much, patience controls emotion, concentration on one thing, over-anxiety, strong determination, less social ability to control deep emotional sadness, emotional shock, over sensitivity to small details.	Anemia due to poor nutrition and digestion; blood stagnation and poor circulation in the hips and legs; feels like fainting, heaviness in the legs, malfunctioning of the intestinal organs, easily fatigued in the hip area, lumbago and sciatica due to curvature in lumbar vertebrae, lack of strength in the hara, poor circulation, blood stagnation, appendicitis; constipation and pain in the side of the cervical vertebrae after appendectomy; hearing difficulty, eye fatigue, abnormal menstrual cycle, pain in the ovaries, stiffness in inner leg, shoulder pain, migraine headaches, pain in back of ears.
	Jitsu	Patient, strong determination to the end, ability to hold everything in himself, accomplishes what he sets out to do, restless, overwork, tendency not to eat slowly, restless rapid eye movements, headaches.	Stiffness in the cervical vertebrae like morning-stiff, difficulty in rotation, puffiness in eyes and ears, feeling of being chilled and hot in the head; redness in the cheek, stiffness in the solar plexus, stiffness and coldness in the lower hara, frequent trips to the toilet, poor circulation in the extremities, frost-bite, poor digestion, constipation, ovary malfunctioning, poor circulation in the legs due to malfunction of the intestinal artery near navel, lower backache due to curvature in the lumbar vertebrae area, pain in the shoulders, pain in the upper part of the teeth, lack of saliva secretion.

Kidney and Bladder Meridians—Function of Endocrine Organs and Purification

Function of the Kidney Meridian		Controlling spirit and energy to the body and governing resistance against mental stress via control of internal hormone secretions. Detoxifies and purifies blood preventing acidosis. Right side between second and third lumbar vertebrae manufactures cortisone. Left side between second and third lumbar vertebrae produces urine by purifying the blood.	
		Psychological	Physical
Kidney Meridian		Anxiety, fear, restlessness, nervous, pessimistic, no desire, family stress, lack of patience and determination, hesitant to move, psychosomatic fatigue.	Blackish, dry, puffy skin lacking elasticity; poor circulation in the hips and hara, frequent trips to the toilet; lower backache due to cold or subluxation in the third and fourth lumbar area; malfunctioning of hormone secretions; lack of sleep; abnormal sex life; reproductive organ problems; cracks in the nails; prone to bone fractures; tendency to stumble, stiffness in the hara or torso muscles.
	Jitsu	Impatient, "work-aholic," nervous sensitivity; restless, constant complaining, too much attention to details, lack of determination.	Blackish color in the face, vomiting, blood in the saliva; prone to nose bleeding and fainting; heaviness in the head; inflamed throat; thirsty; poor hearing when drugs are taken, ringing in the ears; stiffness in the back; tightness in the torso muscles, abnormal hormone secretion, densely colored urine, bitterness in the mouth, bad breath; prone to inflammation; fatigue from overwork.
Function of the Bladder Meridian		Related to mid-brain which cooperates with the kidney hormone system and pituitary gland. Also connected to autonomic nervous system that is related to reproductive and urinary organs. At the same time it eliminates the final product of body liquid purification—urine.	
		Psychological	Physical
Bladder Meridian	Kyo	Strained nerves, stiffness and sensitivity in the body; complaining all the time; easily frightened, night sweating, anxiety.	Nasal congestion; heaviness and pain in the eyes; migraine headache on back of head; malfunctioning of autonomic nervous system, oversensitivity; poor circulation especially in hara and legs; frequent urination, chillness in the back; tendency to bend the back; subluxation in the fifth lumbar vertebra area; tightness in the legs, tension in the hara malfunctioning of the womb; inflammation of the bladder and pain and feeling of retained urine.
	Jitsu	Worry over trivial details; nervous stress; restlessness; oversensitivity.	Stiff-necked pain in lower cervical and thoracic vertebrae. Heaviness in the back of the head towards the eyes. Tension in the shoulder muscles; tightness in the back of the leg; nasal congestion; frequent urination; inflammation or pain in the bladder or prostrate area. Strained autonomic nervous system.

Heart Constrictor and Triple Heater Meridians—Circulatory and Protective Functioning

Function of the Heart Constrictor Meridian		Supplemental function of the heart related to circulatory system including heart sac, cardiac artery; system of arteries and veins. Also controls total nutrition as well as circulation.	
		Psychological	Physical
Heart Constrictor Meridian	Kyo	Restless but immobile; absent-minded; lack of sleep and frequent dreaming; palpitations and shortness of breath, squeezing sensation around the chest.	Difficulty in swallowing; prone to tonsillitis, malfunctioning of the heart organ, strong palpitations, easily fatigued; low blood pressure; dropsy, poor circulation, pain in the stomach and duodenum; abnormal blood pressure, pain in the chest and rib cage.
	Jitsu	Restless when asleep or awake, nervous in social situations, abnormal concentration on work, abnormal emotions, hypersensitivity.	Strong palpitations; high blood pressure; dizziness, easily fatigued; poor circulation; headache; stiffness in the solar plexus; tightness in the hara area; pain in the stomach; cardiac malfunctioning, tingling in the fingers; feverish palms; colitis due to diarrhea or constipation; coated tongue.
Function of the Triple Heater Meridian		Supplemental function of the small intestine. Also controls spirit and visceral organs circulating energy to entire body. Protects function of lymphatic system. Upper heat related to chest, middle heat to solar plexus, heat above the navel and below related to peritoneum and intestinal peritoneum as well as circulation to the extremities.	
		Psychological	Physical
Triple Heater Meridian	Kyo	Mental obsessions; pampered when he was a child, headaches; ringing in the ears; heaviness and dizziness in the head; sensitive to heat, cold and dampness.	Weak mucus tissues and lymphatic system; prone to tonsillitis, nasal problems; swollen lymphatic glands of the cervical vertebrae; sensitive to humidity and temperature change, easily catches cold; tired eyes; sensitive skin; allergic, dizziness in the head; tightness in the chest and hara; liquid stagnation in the hara; abnormal blood pressure, tendency for whiplash conditions to worsen, pain in back of head and temples, abnormal cervical vertebrae.
	Jitsu	Extremely cautious, hypertense, tendency to clench the palms, tightness in the arms, heaviness in the head, nervous reaction to external changes in heat, cold, humidity, heaviness in chest (upper heater) stomach (middle heater) and lower hara.	Overly cautious, sensitive, unconscious tension in the arms, stagnation in the brain causing heavy feeling; abnormal eye pressure; pain in the neck, shoulder, and arms. Lymphatic inflammations; imflammation of nasal mucus skin, prone to inflammations; itchy skin, tightness in the chest, poor circulation in the legs, pain in the rib cage, loose gums, susceptible to humidity, ticklish, inflammation in the mouth and womb; rash.

Liver and Gall Bladder Meridians—Storage and Displacement Function

Function of the Liver Meridian		Stores nutrients and energy for physical activity. Also cultivates resistance against disease and supplies, analyzes, and detoxifies blood to maintain physical energy.	
		Psychological	Physical
Liver Meridian	Kyo	Lack of determination; irritable, easily upset, short-tempered, inconsistent, nevous sensitivity; inability to gain weight, attention to trivial matters.	Weak joints, easily fatigued due to lack of energy; dizziness, tendency to stumble, tired eyes, sees everything in yellow, body's system easily poisoned because of poor detoxification mechanism, fever, no appetite, stiff muscle, lack of sexual energy, impotence, prostrate problems.
	Jitsu	Hard worker, concentrator, stubborn, tendency never to give up. Works impatiently and impulsively until exhausted. Easily affected emotionally, sometimes screams in loud voice, displays emotion and then controls it. Good eater.	Accumulated fatigue due to never ending drive; overeating; excessive drinking, swollen chest and stomach, headaches, heaviness in the head; poor digestion, lack of exercise; dizziness due to lack of blood, high fever without cause, chillness, coughing, liver organ malfunctioning, pulling the anal area causing hemorrhoids, prostrate problems, sensation of the testicles; inflammation of the female reproductive organs, excess of sugar and alcohol, strong movements; pain in the sacrum and coccyx, total stiffness. Tightness in the hara area feeling like a rubber board, flatulence, putrefaction, prone to inflammations.
Function of the Gall Bladder Meridian		Distributes nutrients and balances total energy through the aid of internal hormones and secretion such as bile, saliva, gastric acid, insulin, and intestinal hormones.	
		Psychological	Physical
Gall Bladder Meridian	Kyo	Emotional excitement resulting in hypersensitivity. Sudden fatigue after tension, timid, easily frightened, lack of determination, strained nerves, light sleeper, lack of energy, general fatigue, and no guts.	Tired eyes, no energy due to fatigue caused by improper distribution of nutrients. Tired legs, dull eyes, weak eyesight, lack of bile, poor digestion of fats; prone to get diarrhea and constipation; neuralgia; dizziness, mucus formation in the eyes, pale complexion, anemic, obese in spite of poor appetite, accumulation of fatty tissues without consumption of greasy foods; easily fatigued, gastric hyperacidity, improper nutritional distribution.
	Jitsu	Assumes too much responsibility, fatigued, tendency to push himself in work, pays attention to small details, easily upset, impatient, always in a hurry for nothing; tired eyes, too much concentration.	Lack of sleep causing tired eyes, bloated stomach, loss of appetite, glassy eyes, yellowish in white part of eye and skin; pain, tearing and high pressure in the eyes; tendency to blink frequently, stiffness in the extremities, stiff muscles, pain in the rib cage, bitter taste in the mouth, burning sensation in the chest; gallstones and spasms in the gall bladder, shoulder pain, heaviness in the head, migraine headache, constipation, mucus stagnation, itching in the area of the tonsils, coughing, excessive intake of sweets, lack of sour food consumption.

Experiments Related to the Meridian and Tsubo

In psychology there is an experiment for so-called "threshold value" in which we can discover the sensation received when two distant points are touched. Open the edge of a compass and place both edges on the skin at different points, applying the same amount of pressure to each one. If the points are fairly far apart, you can feel two distinct points. However, when the distance between the points is lessened, you may feel one point instead of two. This is what we call threshold value. This means that at a certain distance between two points you feel one point instead of the two. This varies depending on what part of the skin is touched. For example, on the tip of the tongue, the threshold value is 1 millimeter, lips 5 millimeters, fingertips 7 millimeters, cheeks 11 millimeters, forehead 23 millimeters, posterior of the arms 31 millimeters, anterior of the arms 40 millimeters, back 68 millimeters. When two points are touched on an area of the body at its designated threshold value, you will feel only one point. By understanding the threshold value of a particular part of the body, you will find that the areas with the greatest threshold value are the least sensitive parts of the body.

In a visual context the smaller the threshold value—which in this case means the distance between two objects is clearly distinguished—the better the eyesight. The eyesight chart was developed from this principle. Letters and circles are arranged from the biggest to the smallest consecutively. In other words, to sense visually and to sense tactically involves the ability to sense two points clearly. Initial comprehension of this idea left me stunned. This two-point sensory theory was puzzling but at the same time fascinating. Many psychologists have tried to explain this phenomenon scientifically but have failed. This, however did not stop me from finding my own answer.

The conditioned use of our senses is closely associated with our fundamental life activities which utilize our primal senses. In order to tell the shape of an object, its character and quality, we use our conditioned sense. This also holds true in the two-point sensory theory. Our primal senses, on the other hand, come into play when we feel sensations from the internal organs in forms such as smell and pain. Dr. A. Head's theory called Head's Zone Theory, designates specific areas on the skin that indicate internal organ malfunctioning. According to this theory, our cutaneous nerves are grouped in the same way as those of a fetus. In the production of nerve fibers, the original nerves that are reformed become primal senses while the new nerve fibers become conditioned senses.

Sensing something on the skin is biological, but even primal senses such as that of hearing can also be conditioned sense. For example, when you hear a foreign language for the first time, this is sensed as simple sound, without meaning. But after studying that foreign language and learning the meanings of its sounds, it becomes a tool of communication. This means that your hearing sense is developed in stages. I will give you another example. You believe someone is speaking a foreign language and you are trying to understand it, when suddenly you realize that what you are hearing is your mother tongue spoken with a strange accent. With this recognition his speech can be clearly sensed. The trained sense belongs to new nerve fibers biologically. However, in order to make clear distinctions for analysis and meaning we need the help of consciousness, which comes from the new cerebral cortex system. So through our trained senses we can also discover our primal senses.

Two-point Pressure Experiment

Let's experiment. Hold someone's arm gently with both hands. It doesn't matter whether he is wearing clothes or not, though wearing none may help to get a clearer response. The person should pay no attention to his arm because this is an experiment in skin sensitivity. Any kind of visual stimuli is prohibited. Place one thumb on his arm and then put the other thumb on the same muscle at a distance of more than 50 millimeters. Press a little bit with both thumbs, being careful not to press hard in order to keep the sensation on the conditioned level. (Remember that pain is sensed on the primal level.) On the forearm, the ratio is 40 millimeters, therefore, you can feel these two points as two points because more than 40 can be sensed as two. Then without easing up on your pressure, bring your mind to your hara instead of in the fingertips. When you have done this, you will be in a state of muscular tonus. Muscular tonus is the condition in which the muscle is in a relaxed but prepared state of activity. For example, when you hold a brief case or a bag you are not conscious you are holding that object. You just hold it and sometimes you forget you are holding it but you never drop it. When you are standing up, you do not sense that you are pressing the floor in order to stand. You simply support yourself, without consciousness, in the state of muscular tonus.

But let's go back to the experiment. Without shifting your consciousness to the fingertips, keep youself in a state of muscular tonus. The person whose arm you are touching will feel these two points as one. This doesn't mean your senses have dulled. Press the thumbs again, this time with your consciousness. He will feel clearly two pressure points. Once more completely relax and place yourself in the state of muscular tonus. He may again feel the two points as only one. I believe this experiment is fundamental in order to sense the tsubos and the meridian lines. So you have to try until you succeed. If you fail, try his other arm, or legs, in order to limit his awareness of the experiment. Or ask somebody to try this experiment on you. The subject must be completely relaxed and unself-conscious. Most failures come from the practitioner. The more experienced he is, the more he feels failure. Because he believes in shiatsu, he has a tendency to press with his thumbs. In Japanese sword way (*kendo*) an amateur holds the sword with tensed fingertips. The master holds his sword with his hara. Even when he swings the sword, he swings his body from hara. He can get great *Ki* energy from his body.

How to Use Your Hara

When you concentrate all your energy in your hara, in two-hand shiatsu, the patient feels oneness with you in the deep of his body. Shiatsu with one thumb on top of the other cannot achieve this sensation of oneness, because there is too much tension in the fingertips to utilize the tsubo. In order to tell an amateur from a professional, I ask them to show me two-point shiatsu technique. Unskilled practitioners blindly concentrate on the fingertips. A master gives *Ki* energy from the hara, in a state of complete relaxation. If you complain that your shiatsu isn't achieving good results after hard study in this field, please experiment with this theory. I guarantee you that you will change.

Until recently, I didn't know this convenient and effective method. I had been emphasizing a "both hands," "yin and yang," "tonification-sedation" method for years, but I couldn't discover the difference between two-point shiatsu and one-point shiatsu. I happened to discover this method from my students when I was lecturing.

My psychological training gave me an unconscious hint about this technique. Concentration from hara and relaxation of the whole body is natural. All Japanese culture is based on this principle. If you tighten your shoulders or extremities, your movement becomes clumsy and awkward. Training in the arts is simply how to eliminate this distorted tension. When your movement starts floating naturally, without any tension, real beauty comes out. Also in sports, like *sumo* (Japanese wrestling), you have to use your hara, instead of your hands. In baseball, instead of straining to throw the ball perfectly, use your hara. You have to play baseball naturally, without desire. So, in shiatsu, don't depend on fingertip technique. Instead train yourself to feel the energy flowing within yourself.

Life-compassion

After you attain this two-as-one sensation, put one thumb on a different meridian. You cannot immediately get two-as-one consciousness because you are applying two hands on two different meridians. But if you stay there, gradually two-as-one sensations will come. If you train more carefully, you can achieve a primitive feeling of oneness with the patient. Your two thumbs can feel as one. "One" doesn't mean as if they were on top of each other. Between your two thumbs you can feel a sort of echo or spark, and then they feel as one through the patient, like a circle. You can create oneness or compassion with the patient by using two hands. At the same time the patient can feel the two-as-one sensation. We call this sharing "life-compassion." Life can be maintained only through this sense ef connection. Our single life doesn't exist independently or scattered, but survives as a whole. Life cannot be separated from its environment. Life separates to increase. This doesn't mean life is divided. In the evolution of life, each life evolves a little from its origin. What the division into male and female means is that the unifying of male and female creates new life. Since ancient times the question of what life is has preoccupied science. This is a study about life. The sensation of life is, I believe, the sensation of two-as-oneness. When you feel oneness there is life. When we are completely healthy, we feel oneness with our bodies. On the contrary, when we are unhealthy, stomach, head, arms, and legs are separated and are felt as foreign. If you take care of your stomach, it can be you. But when you ignore it, the stomach will insist on its existence. Because of severe pain in the extremities, people sometimes want to amputate their extremities. But then they cannot be you. If you are used to wearing favorite clothes, they become part of you. Couples and families are the same. If you lose this oneness among your family members, you may notice differences between you and them, rather than their problems, and conflict can result. When lovers need to be one with each other, their life-energy flows. To feel life is to become one and when you feel oneness there is life. The term of "oneness" which I use now is the state of unconsciousness. This is not just a word. This is life-compassion.

The Sensation of Shaking Hands

When lovers hold hands, they not only hold physical hands, but they also feel their spiritual selves. We can feel the other's spirit through shaking hands. In a modern society, we are prone to deal with material things instead of life-spirit. The more you emphasize materialism, the more life-spirit deteriorates. The attitude towards things endangers nature. Pollution is one of the examples. The same thing happens in the human body. Distinguishing consciousness takes place in the new cerebral cortex system. The more the new cerebral cortex system functions, the more the lymphatic system deteriorates, along with the primal sense. The more civilized the people are, the more dull their life-sensations become. Not only these sensations, but also the life-control system can suffer, for more nutrition goes to the new cerebral cortex system and less nutrition goes to the lymphatic system. The more the new cerebral cortex system functions, the less life-maintenance system functions. Thus the more civilized we are the more we are alienated from a healthy life. In our daily routine we have to re-establish this primitive consciousness in order to rejuvenate our lives.

It is an *instinctive* feeling and desire that adds zeal to civilized people's love affairs, to sports, and to social life, for we know that excitement of life-compassion is essential. Without this understanding, people who pursue superficial desires can miss fundamental life fulfillment. In modern life we overemphasize material things, therefore we have less life-compassion. Once you've realized that this life-compassion is essential, you don't need to be crazy for more and stronger stimulants. I believe the popularity of Yoga and Zen in the West arises from this phenomenon. Fundamentally in the East, we emphasize life and life-compassion culture. We don't like to emphasize materialistic life. This is the main reason eastern countries were underdeveloped materially and were slow to establish modern nations. Today the West has discovered that we have life-consciousness in the East and is seeking it. (Some scholars have even explored scientifically the physiological benefits of Zen.) We in the East need to encourage this life-compassion culture in our societies.

What Are Meridians and Tsubo?

The main reason why I discovered some meridians differ from those presented in the classic books is that I followed my intuitive process honestly, by touching. Also, depending on how you stimulate a tsubo, you can get different results. This gives me a different constellation of meridian lines. Another reason may be that I have studied psychology and have had psychological research done on skin and touching mechanisms. Moreover, I have studied the oriental philosophy of life. Meridians and tsubos belong to the most primitive life-function, so the study of meridians and tsubos is the most basic study of life. Even though we comprehend physical life from an anatomical, biochemical point of view, the constitution of life itself is beyond science. You may research meridians and tsubos, and their phenomenal mechanisms with conventional methods, but this approach will be far away from the essential truth. Religion is not intellectual understanding, but practice, because religion deals with life. As you can research Zen from a biological point of view, you can research religion from the point of view of expediency. However, in order to comprehend religion, first you must believe. Through thousands of years, practitioners of oriental medicine have proved the effectiveness of meridians and tsubos, and in order to utilize them we don't need concrete, objective research. So-called masters comprehend without thinking, but enforced explanations give us more chaotic answers, like Zen *koans*. Moreover, artisans, unlike scholars, can be better at their skill. Therefore, it makes scientific explanation more difficult. The reason why meridians and tsubos are important to maintain life and treat disease is because they are life itself. Without life, meridians and tsubos cannot function. Without conscious attention to life-energies, and techniques, you cannot get good result from treatment. No textbook can tell you how to do this, because we are dealing with life itself, beyond words. When the whole life is distorted, meridians and tsubos can not just be pointed to because they show the abnormal phenomena. A sensitive person will notice these phenomena in the form of skin changes, but in order to correct the abnormality, we need life functioning. So what I'm saying here is that in order to understand meridians and tsubos, we must first feel inner life. Life itself is the cure of the disease. Also, the trust that we can cure disease by life is most essential.

3. Basic Techniques of Zen Shiatsu Therapy

How to Tonify and Sedate

The movement of our thumbs and four fingers in such a way inherent only to man allows us to feel the world around us. We feel by grasping, holding, pinching, and supporting. In shiatsu we should be able to instinctively utilize the total mobility of our hands according to nature's laws.

Proper use of both the thumbs and fingers is of utmost importance in administering good shiatsu. Just as the harmony of a democratic government can be disturbed if changed into a dictatorship, the use of the thumbs alone can disturb our body's natural balance. Swollen thumbs, shoulder pain, and resulting fatigue should not be part of the learning process in shiatsu.

In shiatsu we usually employ the use of three fingers. However, we should keep in mind the total strength of all the fingers, including the little fingers.

In ampuku (shiatsu on the abdomen) therapy, pressure given directly on this area of the body is concentrated in the three fingertips, but the main source of strength should come from the wrists, with the thumb relaxed.

Rikyu, founder and master of the Tea Ceremony, once said

> Don't shake your tea whisk with your fingertips,
>   but with your elbow.

I advise my students not to use the strength from the fingertips alone but from your elbows. This is one of the keys to successful shiatsu.

Palm Technique

Noted for its soothing penetration, this is the most widely used technique in shiatsu. In a properly balanced position, the practitioner can apply pressure using his body's weight without causing any damage to the torso or internal organs.

The palms and fingers should be relaxed at all times and hold themselves to the part of the body being treated. For example, if you are treating the back, the hand should rest flat against the body; if you are doing the buttock area, the hand should follow the contour of that area.

You can adjust the amount of pressure exerted in accordance with the distribution of body weight in the "push-up" position. To exert effective but comfortable pressure, the palms remain relaxed on the body, while the arms support your body weight. The angle of your body in relation to your arms will determine the amount of pressure being applied to the patient. It is important that the practitioner remain

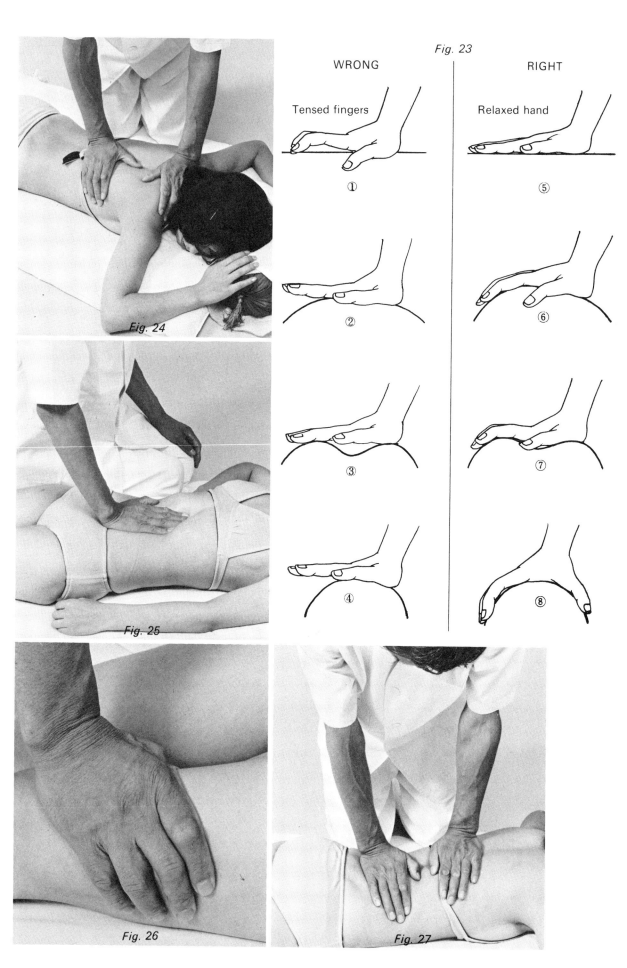

Fig. 23

WRONG | RIGHT

Tensed fingers

Relaxed hand

① ⑤

② ⑥

③ ⑦

④ ⑧

Fig. 24

Fig. 25

Fig. 26

Fig. 27

relaxed. The feeling of pressure on the body should resemble the pull of gravity—natural, effective, but unobtrusive. The kneeling position is employed when light pressure is needed. The closer you kneel next to the patient, the easier it is to exert light pressure. Arms should remain outstretched, hands placed vertically on the patient's body, shoulders slightly forward (Fig. 28).

When a child playfully crawls on someone's back, she is unintentionally applying good shiatsu pressure. The energy of her being is fully concentrated in every movement, and the child's feeling of sincerity in her act penetrates into your body as a healing force. This type of spontaneity and presence should be transferred to your patient with each touch. It is only when the ego is surrendered, that mere pressure on the body becomes a supporting vital force toward health.

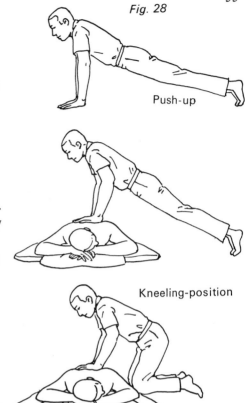

Fig. 28

Push-up

Kneeling-position

Make sure that the patient lies on the stomach flat.

Palm Technique Using Both Hands: Place both palms on the patient and apply pressure over both palms. Proceed down the body by shifting your weight to one hand resting in its original position while sliding the other hand down (Figs. 29 and 30). Redistribute the weight evenly between the two hands. Repeat until the entire area is treated. In performing this movement, neither hand loses contact with the patient's body. The stationary hand tonifies while the active hand sedates.

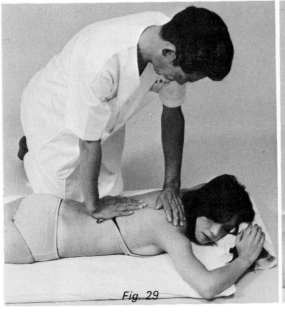

Fig. 29

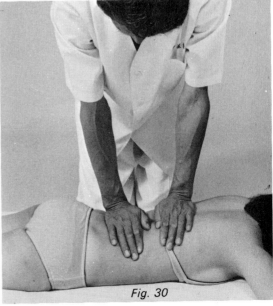

Fig. 30

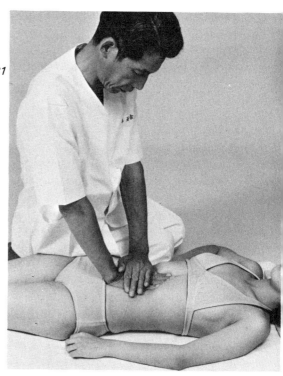

Fig. 31

Palm Technique Using Crossed Hands:
Place one palm on top of the other forming a cross, pressure can be applied with
this technique (Fig. 31).

Undulation Technique: Place both hands, palm down, on the abdomen (*Hara* in
Japanese) and in one continuous motion, shift the pressure from your four fingers to
your palms in a wavelike motion. This technique relaxes and comforts the hara area
and its deeper organs (Fig. 32).

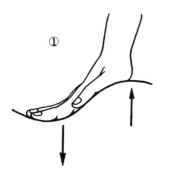

Fig. 32

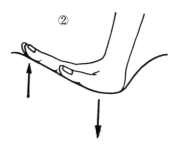

Fig. 33

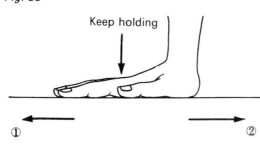

Keep holding

Vertical Pressure: Apply pressure with
your palm perpendicular to the body.
Vibrating the palms help relax the area
being treated (Fig. 33).

Circular Massage: Apply light pressure using a circular movement. This technique is especially good for relaxing the muscles surrounding the shoulder blades (Fig. 34).

Fig. 34

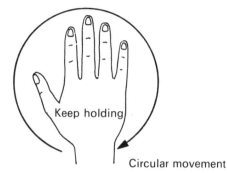

Keep holding

Circular movement

Rub Down Technique: While applying pressure to an area of the body, you can "rub down" the muscle. This technique is different from regular massage in that the hand slides along the muscle in a vertical position.

Grasping Technique: Hold your patient's body as if you were shaking hands or holding something and apply steady pressure (Figs. 35 and 36). The patient can receive pleasant sensations when the proper tsubo-points are pressed.

Fig. 35

Fig. 36

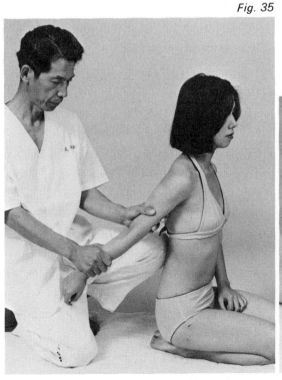

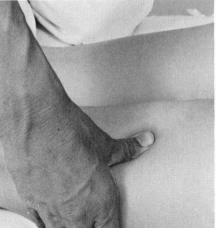

58

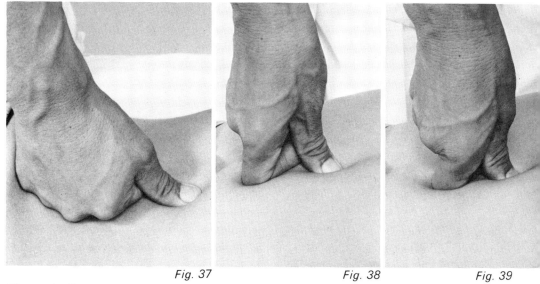

Fig. 37   Fig. 38   Fig. 39

Fingertip Pressure

When using the tip of your thumb, extend your other fingers outward in order to support your thumb. Your thumb should not carry the entire burden of weight. There are many techniques for using your fingertips as seen in Figs. 37–43. The technique you use should depend on the area you are treating as well as comfortability and convenience from your position. In order to reach narrow areas in between bones or muscles, you can apply pressure with the nail area. Because sensitive nerves are concentrated in the nail area, the flow of the meridians can be easily detected using this technique.

When diagnosing the hara area, all the fingertips can be used.

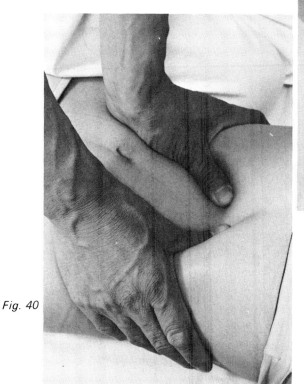

Fig. 41

Fig. 40

Thumb Pressure: Extend the thumb and make a fist with the other four fingers. Thumb and four fingers together, apply pressure with the thumb and fist area between the second and third finger joints (Fig. 37). I also use the thumb supported by four extended fingers. The thumb sedates while the four fingers tonify (Fig. 40).

Four Finger Pressure: With your four fingers together, apply pressure. Strength should come from the elbows and palms with thumb relaxed (Fig. 41).

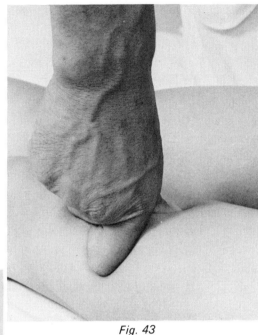

Fig. 43

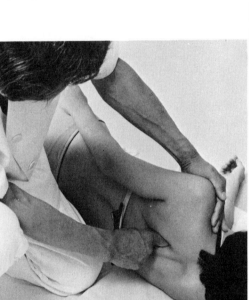

Fig. 42

Pressure Applied with Three Fingers: You can apply pressure using three fingers in the same manner as four fingers. This technique is often used in diagnosing the hara area.

Two Finger Technique: With the index finger bent supporting the thumb, apply pressure with both the thumb (to tonify) and the second joint of the index finger (to sedate) (Fig. 42).

Two Finger Pinching Technique: You can lightly pinch the area being treated before applying pressure (Fig. 43).

Remember that when you are applying any of the fingertip techniques, you are using both hands simultaneously. One hand should act as a stabilizing force that supports your body's weight when the other hand moves from one point to the next. In this case, the supporting hand, which is placed on the body palm down, tonifies (yin), while the other hand using the fingertips sedates (yang) (Fig. 44). The total pressure applied by both palm and fingertips should be comfortable but firm enabling the patient to remain relaxed and open to the benefits of the treatment.

Because little movement is involved in this type of technique, the practitioner can conserve his energy, avoid fatigue, and concentrate on feeling the energy flow within his patient.

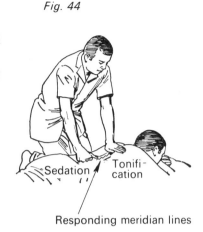

Fig. 44

Sedation   Tonification

Responding meridian lines

Three Rules Governing Shiatsu

(1) *Vertical Pressure*

Firm pressure applied vertically on the body promotes good health. Though nonvertical pressure promotes good blood circulation, it can damage the natural healing force within the body particularly in the case of illness.

(2) *Stationary Pressure*

Pressure applied without movement is essential in giving good shiatsu. The length of time to hold each point varies from 2–7 seconds, but there are cases where 8–30 seconds is needed. Pressure applied in such a way penetrates into the body, stimulating the parasympathetic nervous system which in turn calms the internal organs and body as a whole.

(3) *Supporting Pressure*

When we stand, sit, or move, the structure of our body remains in balance with the aid of our muscles. We are not conscious of our muscles contracting or expanding, yet they are there to support and maintain us structurally. It is this feeling of support that we transfer through our touch. The Japanese character meaning human is written 人. The two lines can represent two human beings supported by each other. This type of relationship should exist between patient and practitioner. The patient and practitioner interrelate, supporting and exchanging their energies throughout the treatment. If you give shiatsu to someone whose muscles are tense and not relaxed, no amount of pressure will penetrate his body. Therefore, it is necessary that pressure coming from one direction be supported by something from the opposite direction. When a person lies flat on the floor during a shiatsu treatment, the floor acts as the supporting force to the pressure being exerted by the practitioner. In two-hand manipulation, supporting pressure is given because one hand sedates while the other tonifies.

Two-hand Manipulation

From the eastern point of view, all living things are governed by opposing forces called yin and yang. It is close interaction and harmony between these two forces that constitute a balanced healthy body. In Japanese we call the yin force *kyo* and the yang force *jitsu*. We deal with *kyo* through tonification, *jitsu* through sedation. When our energy flows (meridians) become unbalanced or stagnated, sickness results.

In two-hand manipulation we follow the *kyo-jitsu* principle in which one hand assumes the supportive or yin role and the other hand the active or yang role. By working with these two forces simultaneously, we can promote balanced energy flow in the body. Acupuncture employs the same principle in selecting the type of metal used for their needles. The composition of one needle may be minus (yin) while the other plus (yang).

An essential aspect of mastering two-hand manipulation is understanding the importance of the supporting hand (yin). When we observe a magician performing a trick we are attracted to the hand in motion. However, it is the stationary hand that actually performs the trick. In shiatsu, the supportive (yin) hand provides penetrating support needed to prepare the body for treatment. Without this force, the manipulation with the hand in motion (yang) will remain superficial and often painful. The interaction between the *kyo* and *jitsu* forces utilizing two-hand manipulation is the only way toward an effective method of balancing our body's energy flow.

Manipulation

Shiatsu is one of two systems of manipulation, the other is *Seitai* or structural realignment. Old style anma (Japanese massage) consists of *ankyo* and the so-called Do-In method.

In shiatsu, both pressure and manipulation should be used to complement each other. In this case, applied pressure acts as the *kyo* element while manipulation acts as *jitsu*.

Other forms of manipulation include *Katsu* (emergency survival techniques), chiropractics, osteopathy, and physical therapy.

Isometrical exercise and medical massage methods aim at rehabilitating muscle strength.

In my shiatsu treatments, I usually combine pressure and manipulative techniques to obtain a more accurate diagnosis of the body's overall condition and balance of energy flow. The use of manipulative therapy alone does not penetrate to the fundamental cause of the problem which exists in the energy flow. Therefore, applied shiatsu and ampuku therapy are necessary to provide the fundamental strength needed for the body to heal itself.

Fundamental Concepts in the Use of Manipulation

(1) *Warm-Up*
Warming up the muscles and ligaments by giving applied shiatsu and a gentle rubdown prepares the patient for the treatment that follows. At this time, you çan feel the condition of the muscles, tendons, and ligaments. You can also detect subluxations of the vertebra, dislocated joints and other abnormalities that may exist. The treatment should proceed according to the *kyo-jitsu* principle explained previously.

(2) *Establishing a Center Point for Manipulation*
Before administering any type of manipulation therapy, a center point must be established. This center point acts as the stabilizing point around which the movements revolve. One hand is usually centered on this point enabling the other hand to maneuver the manipulation somewhat effortlessly.

(3) *Utilizing Maximum Stretch*
With one hand supporting the joint or muscle area, rotate or stretch the area to its maximum point of flexibility. Patient should be able to remain comfortable in the position while at the same time feeling the stretch. Hold the position while keeping the patient relaxed. Then move back to the normal position slowly. Muscle tone can increase with the use of this technique and the patient should gain greater mobility in his movements. It is important to remember that this technique should be performed slowly. Sudden thrusts can damage the area instead of revitalize it.

How to Give Total Body Shiatsu

Four Diagonoses in Oriental Medicine

A shiatsu treatment usually begins in the sitting position. However, if the patient is sick, you may begin with the patient in a reclined position.

In order to understand the general condition of the patient, four types of diagnosis are employed:

Bo-shin—diagnosis through general observation (appearance, etc.)
Bun-shin—diagnosis through sounds, listening (voice tone, etc.)
Mon-shin—diagnosis by way of verbal inquiries directed toward the patient
Setsu-shin—diagnosis through the sense of touch

In oriental diagnosis the practitioner seeks an understanding of the patient as a whole being in a similar way when two people encounter each other. First, they observe their appearances, exchange greetings, listen to the tone of each other's voice, notice any particular odor or smell, ask each other questions, and shake hands or embrace.

In western medicine diagnosis is directed more toward the complaint rather than the complainer. Like a detective looking for a criminal, the doctor conducts an investigation to discover the disease afflicting the body without regard for the patient himself. So the patient is treated as a sick object rather than a human being. This type of doctor-patient relationship is considered unnatural in oriental diagnosis.

Respect, trust, and affection for each other as human beings is very important for successful diagnosis. The practitioner should be confident in his skill to heal but at the same time respect and understand his patient. When this type of relationship exists, accurate diagnosis can be achieved.

In diagnosis, you should understand the patient's general condition, whether the patient is *kyo* or *jitsu*, yin or yang, whether the complaint is acute or chronic.

In diagnosis, standing first behind the patient is preferable to starting from the front because it requires that the patient concentrate and understand you through your touch rather than face to face confrontation. The patient will feel relaxed and comfortable in an atmosphere of mutual trust and respect, and diagnosis will proceed more accurately. At this point, you should also notice any distortions or subluxations in the spine's structure as well as the condition and flexibility of the back muscles. When the patient is lying on her back, you should observe the color and expression on her face, ask her how she feels and listen to the way she speaks and the tone of her voice. Also sensing body odor and breath odor, if any, is important. Before asking the patient any specific questions concerning her health, utilize all your knowledge while conducting hara diagnosis. When you ask the patient any questions, close attention should be paid to her reaction and response.

When you finish the diagnostic stage, have the patient remain in a sitting position. If, for some reason she cannot sit up, have her lie on her side. The treatment may then begin.

In administering total body shiatsu we do not have any definite order or procedure to follow. However, a general rule for beginners who cannot clearly diagnose *kyo* and *jitsu* and the meridian lines is to follow the basic idea of tonification and sedation mentioned previously. After mastering this basic technique you will be able to modify it according to the condition of the patient and develop your own style.

Sitting Position

Administering Shiatsu to the Shoulder Blade Area:
Place your right hand, palm down, over the back area from the seventh cervical vertebra to the area governing the heart constrictor meridian (① in Fig. 46). Support the patient by placing your left hand on the patient's shoulder. Apply slight pressure using your body weight to the right hand. Hold for two breaths and coordinate your *Ki* energy with the patient's. Then slide the right hand on the spine. This technique enables you to clearly diagnose the condition of the shoulders, spine, and hips (Fig. 45).

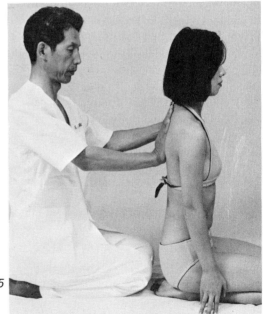

Fig. 45

Fig. 46

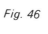

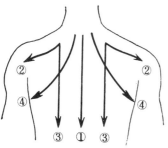

Fig. 47

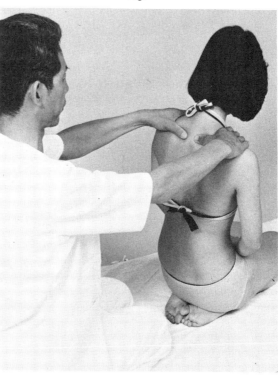

Fig. 48

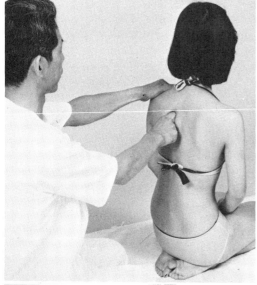

Place both hands on top of the shoulders of the patient. Slide both hands along the shoulder to the shoulder joint (② in Fig. 46) while pressing lightly with the thumbs. Slide back to original position (Fig. 47).

Two-Finger Shiatsu along the Spine: Supporting the patient with your left hand on her left shoulder, give shiatsu down the spine (③ in Fig. 46) using the thumb and bent index finger. Pressure should be applied between the second and eighth thoracic vertebrae, twice on each side (Fig. 48).

Thumb Shiatsu in between Shoulder Blade and Spine: Supporting the patient with your left hand on her left shoulder, place the right hand on her right shoulder so that the thumb rests on the edge of the left shoulder blade (④ in Fig. 46). Slide the thumb underneath the shoulder blade and apply pressure from the top to the bottom of the shoulder blade. Do this twice on each side (Fig. 49).

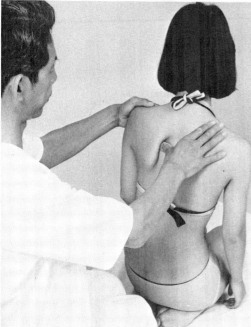

Fig. 49

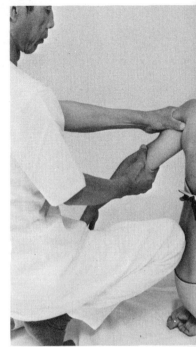

Fig. 50

Upper Arm Shiatsu and Manipulative Exercise Technique:
Support the patient's back on the left side. Holding her left
shoulder with your left hand, bring her left arm backward and
gently apply shiatsu with the four fingers of the right hand in
a squeezing motion from the top of the shoulder to the elbow
(Figs. 50 and 52). Holding the elbow with the right hand,
repeat using the left hand (Fig. 51) Repeat once more alternating hands again and changing the angle of the patient's arm
so that both sides of the arm are treated. Use the same technique covering the area from the elbow to the wrist. Do each
side twice.

Hold the patient's left wrist with your right hand and apply
shiatsu to LI-4, the point located between the thumb and index
finger. Then lightly press and pull the fingers of the patient's
left hand individually using your thumb and index finger.

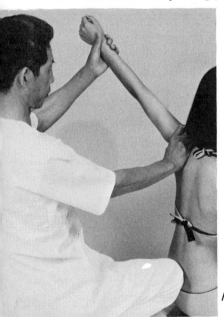

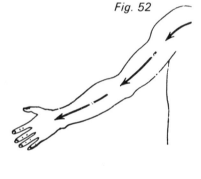

Fig. 52

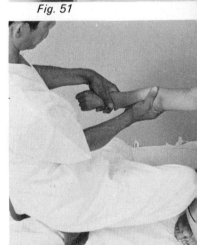

Fig. 51

Fig. 53

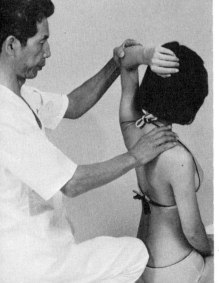

Supporting the patient firmly with your right
hand on her left shoulder, hold her left arm with
your left hand and rotate the patient's arm in as
large a circular motion and slowly as possible (Fig.
53).

Repeat a couple of times on the same side checking muscle tone and the condition of the related
meridians (Fig. 54). Follow the same procedure
with the right arm.

Fig. 54

Fig. 55

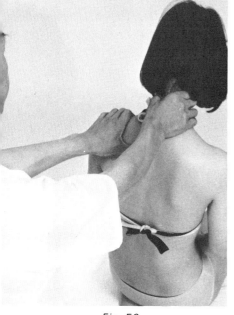

Concentrated Neck Shiatsu and Manipulation: Holding her left shoulder with your left hand, squeeze the patient's neck with your right hand (Fig. 55). Do two–three times on each side. This technique is very good for diagnosing the neck. Be careful not to exert extreme pressure on the jugular vein since this may cause fainting.

With your right hand supporting the base of the skull and the left hand holding her forehead, rotate her head around in as wide a circular motion and slowly as possible. After two rotations change directions and rotate two more times. Then bend her head back and upward stretching her spine with the lifting movement (Fig. 56).

Thumb Shiatsu on the Shoulder Blade: With the four fingers of each hand resting on the patient's shoulders place both thumbs on the top of the shoulder blades on each side (Fig. 57). Apply pressure by standing up and shifting your weight forward, transferring the strength to your arms.

Gradually apply pressure to the top of the shoulders with the thumbs, working from the neck out. You can bend your leg slightly at the knee and let it rest against the back of the patient. You will find this position very comfortable.

Fig. 56

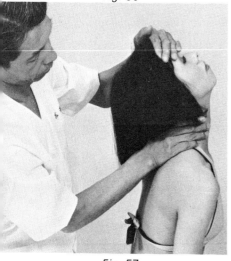

Two Thumb Shiatsu between the Shoulder Blade and Spine: In the standing position, take one step backward and place both thumbs on each side of the spine. Go down the spine (Fig. 58).

Fig. 57

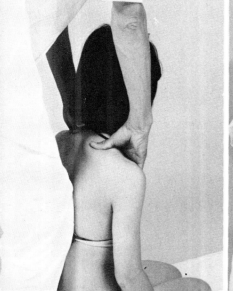

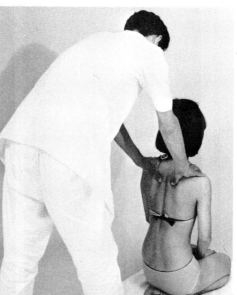

Fig. 58

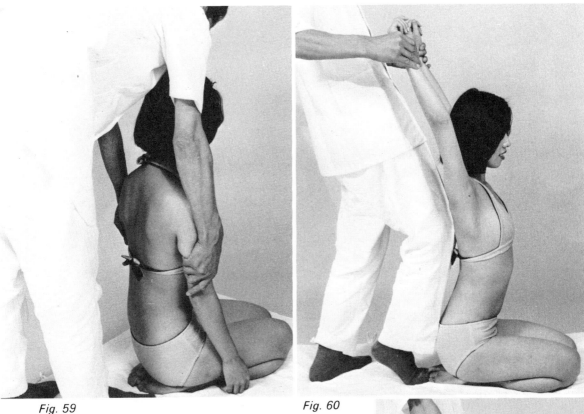

Fig. 59

Fig. 60

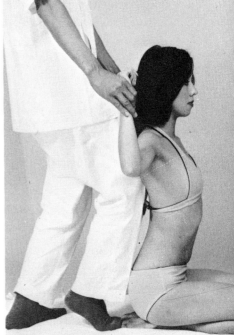

Fig. 61

Upper Arm Manipulation: Holding the patient's shoulders with both hands, apply light shiatsu to the upper arms with your fingers and thumbs a few times (Fig. 59). Then hold her arms securely, rotate them three times using as wide a circular motion as possible (Fig. 60). Support the patient's body by resting your knee against her back. After rotating them, lift both arms straight up and back and stretch the body. With your hands still holding the arms securely, let the arms drop in a relaxed position (Fig. 61). Following this exercise, rub down the back. This technique is very effective in relieving shoulder tension.

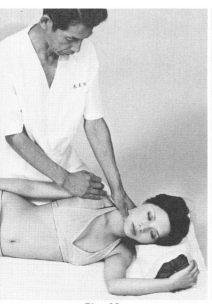

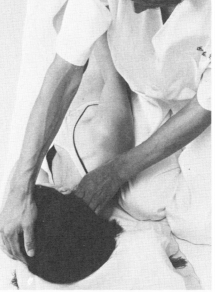

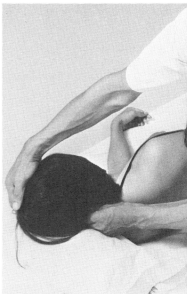

Fig. 62   Fig. 63   Fig. 64

Fig. 65
▶

Shiatsu Applied on the Side Position

Lying on the side is one of the most comfortable positions for the patient to receive shiatsu. It is advisable to lay your patient on the right side first, then on the left side, from the sitting position so that the heart, located on the left side, can remain relaxed. In figures here the patient lies on the right side, in case of the left, do the same procedure. Of course, this procedure depends upon the condition of the patient. As the practitioner, you may find this position a little awkward, but if you support your patient with your body weight instead of merely pressing with your fingers, you can stabilize your position. It is important that the patient remain relaxed in this position.

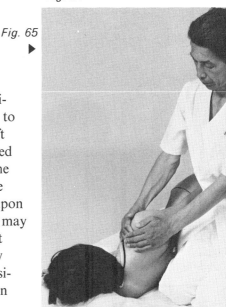

Fig. 66

Neck Shiatsu: With the patient lying on her right side, support her body by placing your left hand on her right shoulder. Give gentle shiatsu to the entire neck area from top to bottom along the meridian lines (Fig. 62).

Front, Side and Back Neck Shiatsu: Supporting your patient's forehead with your left hand, apply two-finger shiatsu along the base of the skull (GB-20, BL-10, and GV–16 area) and hold (Figs. 63 and 64).
    Grasp the patient's right shoulder with both hands and pull down (Fig. 65).

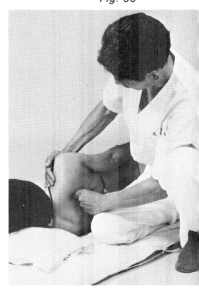

Thumb Shiatsu for Area between Shoulder Blade and Spine: Supporting her shoulder firmly, apply shiatsu with the thumb and bent index finger in the area between the shoulder blade and spine (in the area of the first and eighth thoracic vertebrae). You can also give shiatsu twice around the perimeter of the shoulder blade (Fig. 66).

Upper Arm Holding Technique: Facing the patient's back at a 90 degree angle and supporting her back with both knees, hold her upper arms with both hands and lightly apply shiatsu with the fingers and thumbs (Fig. 67). Rest one hand on the shoulder area and give shiatsu with the other hand from the top of the arm to the elbow and wrists. Then holding her wrist, repeat with the other hand.

Upper Arm Manipulation: Open the patient's hand (Fig. 68) and extend her arm upward so that it rests against your chest, palm facing outward (Fig. 69). Bend backward holding arm securely against chest. Then rotate her arm in as wide a circular motion as possible with one hand holding her wrist and the other placed at the armpit. In rotating her arm, try to touch her arm to her ear (Figs. 70 and 71).

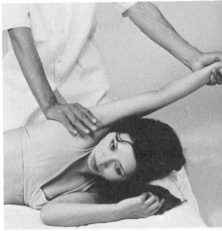

Fig. 70

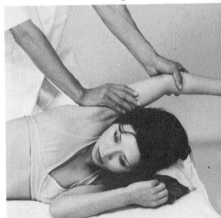

Fig. 71

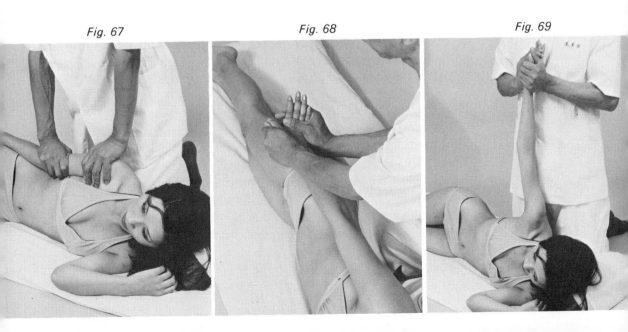

Fig. 67

Fig. 68

Fig. 69

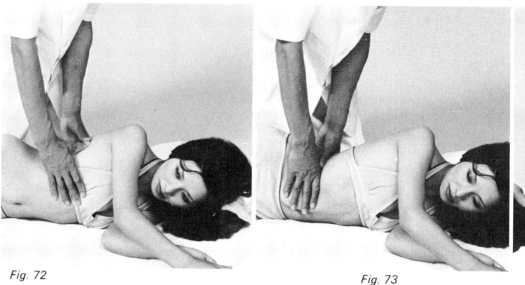

Fig. 72   Fig. 73

Side Shiatsu Using Both Thumbs: With the patient on her side, arm resting in front, give shiatsu on the side from the armpit to the hip using thumbs. Thumbs should press in between the ribs along the gall bladder meridian. This technique is very good for stomach and intestinal problems such as constipation. You must be careful not to damage the rib cage (Figs. 72 and 73).

Two-finger Shiatsu along the Spine: Supporting her rib cage with your right hand, give shiatsu along the spine using your thumb and bent index finger (Fig. 74).

Hip Shiatsu: Move your body so that you face toward the patient's feet. Supporting her body with one hand, give shiatsu to the lower back between the third and fifth lumbar vertebrae, hips and sacrum with two fingers (Fig. 75). Give shiatsu along the small intestine, large intestine, and gall bladder meridians. Use one thumb on top of the other when doing the side of the hips (Fig. 76).

Shiatsu for the Legs: Supporting her hip with one hand, give shiatsu with the other hand to the front and side of the thigh to the knee (Fig. 77). Give gentle shiatsu to the lower leg area with the thumb in back and the four fingers in front down to the ankle (Fig. 78).

Side Shiatsu Adjustment: Supporting the patient's shoulder with your right hand, hold her left knee with your left hand. Place your left knee against her hip and your right knee against her scapula. Lean backwards pulling the shoulder and leg with you stretching her body like a bow (Fig. 79). Return to original position and give shiatsu along the spine with your right hand supporting her shoulder with your left hand. Do a couple of times, change sides and repeat.

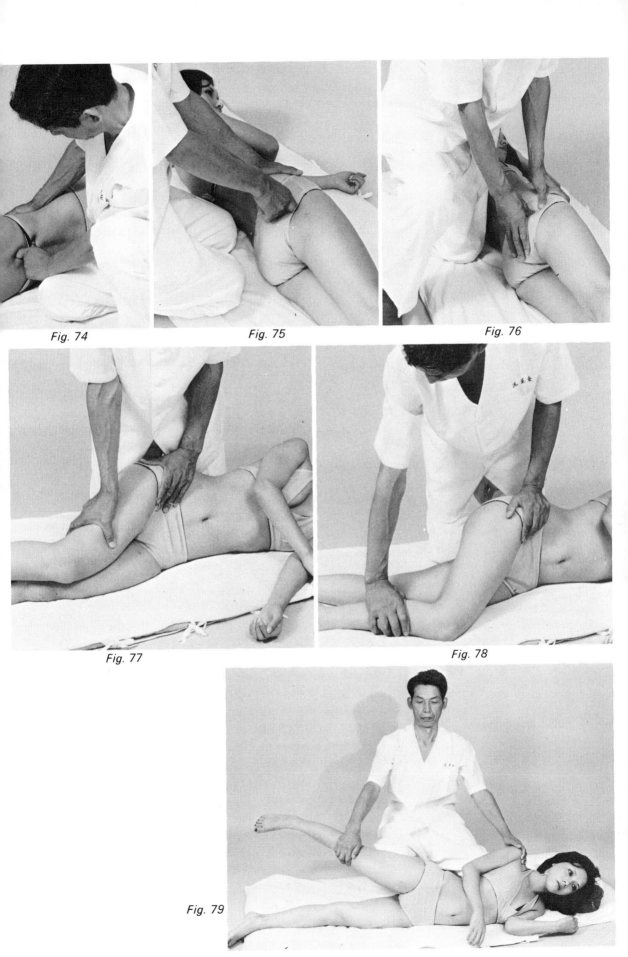

Fig. 74

Fig. 75

Fig. 76

Fig. 77

Fig. 78

Fig. 79

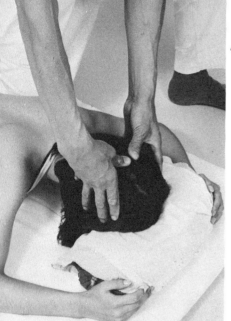

Fig. 80

Lying Down on the Stomach

People suffering from lung or heart problems should avoid using this position. You should also omit this position when treating patients who are uncomfortable lying on their stomach. Instead, give thorough·shiatsu with the patient lying on her side.

Shiatsu for the Back of the Head: Rest her forehead against a firm pillow and give shiatsu down the back of her head with one thumb on top of the other, the four fingers of each hand supporting the side of the head. You can give strong shiatsu along the governing vessel,

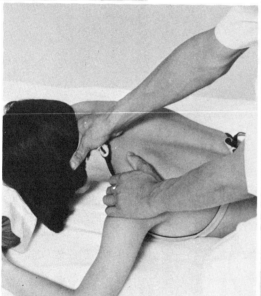 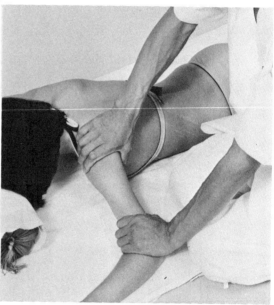

Fig. 81   Fig. 82

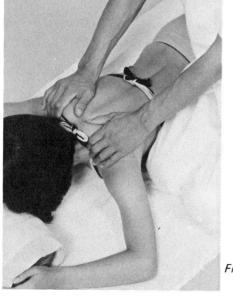

bladder, and gall bladder meridians (Fig. 80). Then grasp her left shoulder with your left hand and pull it downward. With your right thumb give shiatsu to BL-10 and GB-20 areas squeezing the neck gently (Fig. 81).

Support the patient's left shoulder with your right hand. Give gentle squeezing shiatsu to the left upper arm with your left hand (Fig. 82). Repeat the same procedure to opposite side. After completing this technique on both sides, grasp the patient's shoulders, right hand on right shoulder, left hand on left shoulder, and pull shoulders down toward direction of the feet (Fig. 83).

Fig. 83

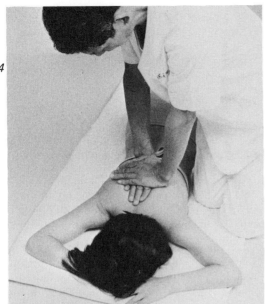

Fig. 84

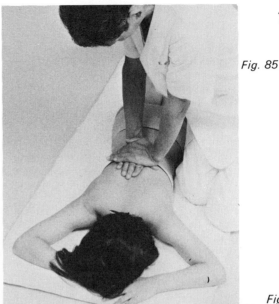

Fig. 85

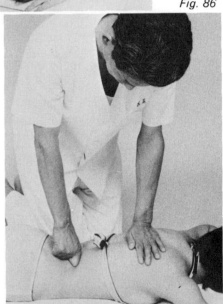

Fig. 86

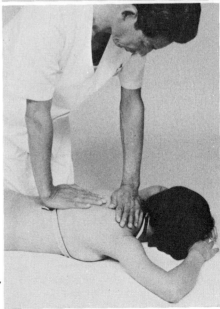

Fig. 87

73

Back Shiatsu: Remove the pillow from under the patient's head and turn her head to the side most comfortable for her. Be sure both shoulders are lying flat on the floor. Gently rub the spine, with your right hand. Then place your left hand on top of your right hand so that the hands form a cross. Give shiatsu with the hands gently as she breathes out, from the top of the spine to the sacrum (Figs. 84 and 85).

Again be sure shoulders are resting completely on the floor. Give shiatsu with her exhalation along the spine with your thumb first on the right side of the spine and then on the left side (Fig. 86). Then go down the spine again gently and slowly with both thumbs on each side of the spine. The area covered should be from first thoracic vertebra to second lumbar vertebra. After you finish this, support the patient with your left hand on seventh cervical vertebra and apply shiatsu on the spine with the heel of your palm. Pressure should be exerted at a 90 degree angle to the spine. In Fig. 87, the palm tonifies while the two fingers sedate.

In using shiatsu techniques avoid strong pressure. Instead concentrate on feeling for any subluxations of the spine and distortions and stiffness in the muscles. *Jitsu* points are very easy to find because they are obviously distorted areas. *Kyo* points are deeper and therefore more difficult to find but more important than the *jitsu* points. In using tonification-sedation techniques, hold the *jitsu* point with one hand and concentrate on tonifying the *kyo* point with the other hand. Once the *kyo* point is tonified, the *jitsu* point will correct itself.

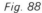
Fig. 88

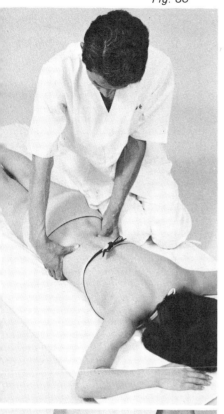

Hip Shiatsu: Strong shiatsu on the back between the second and fourth lumbar vertebrae is potentially harmful because it may cause subluxations of the spine. In this case, place one thumb on each side of the spine and slide both thumbs slowly down the spine to the hips without exerting any pressure (Fig. 88). Check for any subluxations, distortions, or curvatures of the spine.

Place your thumb on the *kyo* point and apply pressure with the palm to the *jitsu* point, which is tight and contracted. Then apply gentle pressure to the *kyo* area (Fig. 89).

When you tonify the *kyo* point through deeper manipulation, you can gradually feel the return of the muscle's elasticity. Support both sides of her spine with your palms and squeeze gently (Fig. 90).

Supporting her hip with your left hand, apply shiatsu with two fingers on the sacrum, small intestine and large intestine meridians on the hip area (Fig. 91).

Fig. 89

Fig. 90

Fig. 91

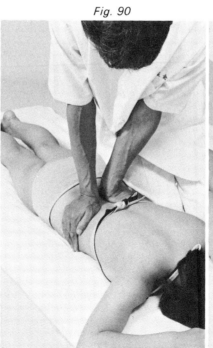

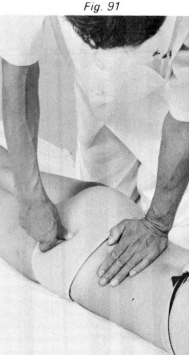

Shiatsu on the Back of the Leg: Supporting the patient's right hip with your left hand, apply shiatsu with your right palm from the bottom of the buttocks to the back of the knee (Fig. 92). Do this twice on each side. Slide your left palm down to support the upper thigh and apply shiatsu to the lower legs of each side (Fig. 93).

Press hard with both fists on the arches of the patient's feet (Fig. 94). Then rub down the patient gently with your palms first from the feet to the knee, then up the thighs to the hips (Fig. 95). Rotate both palms on the buttock area. Then proceed up the spine to the shoulder. Finish shiatsu on the back by supporting her waist with both hands.

Fig. 92

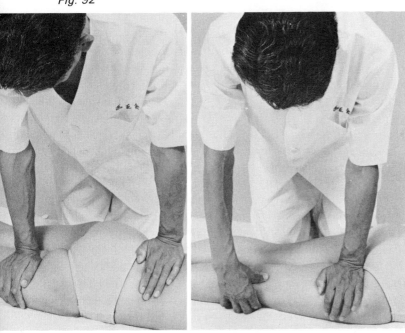

Fig. 93

Fig. 94   *Fig. 95*

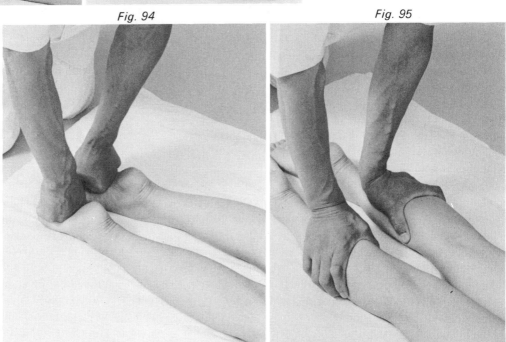

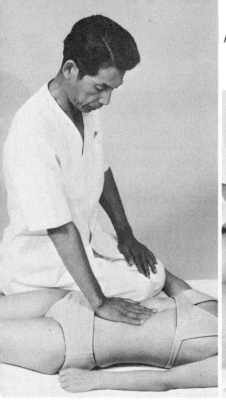

Fig. 96

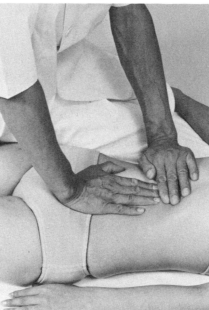

Fig. 97

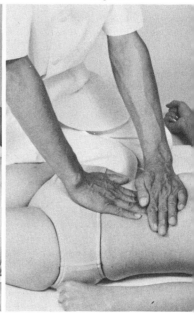

Fig. 98

Supine Position for Shiatsu

During the time when general shiatsu was in vogue among shiatsu practitioners, Shinsai Ota wrote an epoch-making book on shiatsu emphasizing the importance of ampuku or hara (abdomen) therapy. This therapy
was considered so difficult and sophisticated that even nowadays some
practitioners separate it from other techniques by specifically designat-
ing on their office plagues "Anma (Japanese Massage) and Ampuku."
Many shiatsu schools and practitioners as well as patients do not abide
by the theory of ampuku. This may be because of the influence of
western manipulative techniques as well as modern medicine. In any
case, ampuku is a very important part of shiatsu and can contribute
enormously toward helping the critically ill and those patients who require calm but penetrating manipulation. Ampuku therapy not only
allows the patient to remain tranquil, it also rehabilitate the patient's
internal functioning and is an important part of diagnosis. Therefore,
it is important that we do not neglect ampuku therapy. You can begin
with the hara when the patient is in the supine position, do her legs and
then come back up to the neck.

Using the Palm on the Hara Area: Place the three fingers of your right
hand on the solar plexus area, the heel of your palm on the navel and
your thumb and little finger spread out to the side. You can give gentle
pressure with all five fingers while the patient takes two deep breaths
(Figs. 96 and 97).

Fig. 99

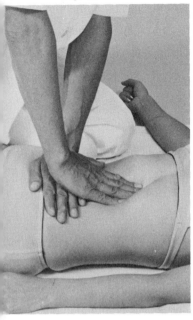

Slide the right hand down to the lower hara and place the left hand palm down, on the upper hara and apply pressure with both hands simultaneously, using your body weight (Fig. 98).

Do the same technique as in Fig. 99, but instead slide the left hand down to the lower hara and place the right hand on the upper hara.

Upper Hara Diagnosis Using Three Fingers: Place your right hand on the lower hara area, and with your three fingers press gently and proceed with diagnosis of the solar plexus area. Solar plexus—heart meridian, artery—heart constrictor meridian, stomach area—stomach meridian, left rib cage—triple heater meridian, gall bladder—gall bladder meridian, right rib cage—liver meridian, left kidney—kidney meridian, left side of hara—bladder meridian, left rib cage—lung meridian, right kidney—kidney meridian, right side of hara—bladder meridian, right rib cage—lung meridian (see Figs. 100–109).

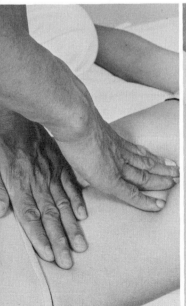

Fig. 100 Heart meridian

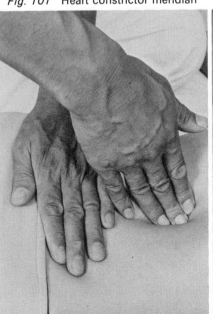

Fig. 101 Heart constrictor meridian

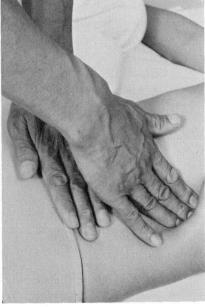

Fig. 102 Stomach meridian

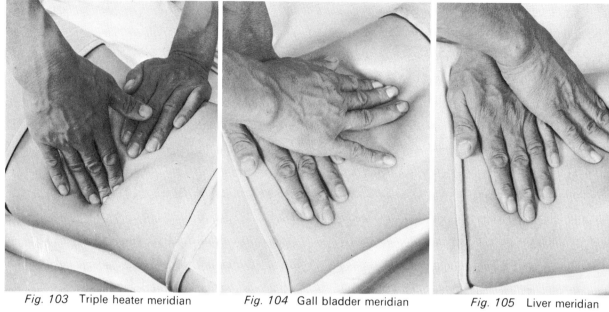

Fig. 103 Triple heater meridian   Fig. 104 Gall bladder meridian   Fig. 105 Liver meridian

Fig. 106
Kidney meridian

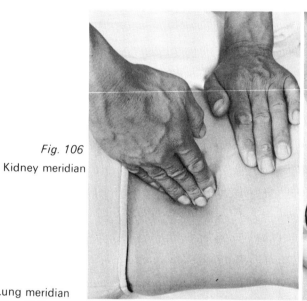

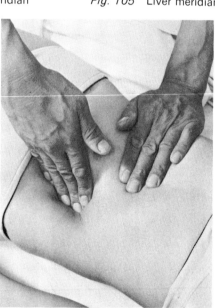

Fig. 108 Lung meridian

Fig. 107
Bladder meridian

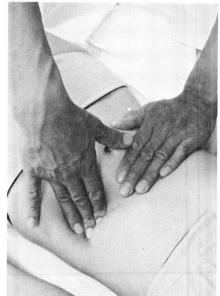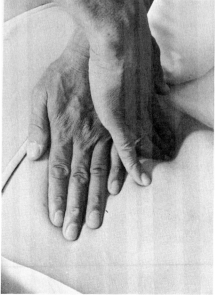

Fig. 109
Lung meridian (right)

Shiatsu to the Lower Hara Using Three Fingers: Supporting the upper part of the hara with your left hand, continue diagnosing with the three fingers of your right hand on these points: navel—spleen meridian, below navel (*tanden*)—kidney meridian, lower hara—bladder meridian, left small intestine—small intestine meridian, left large intestine—large intestine meridian, right small intestine—small intestine meridian, right large intestine—large intestine meridian (see Figs. 110–116). You should be able to feel which points are *kyo* or which points *jitsu*.

Fig. 110
Spleen meridian

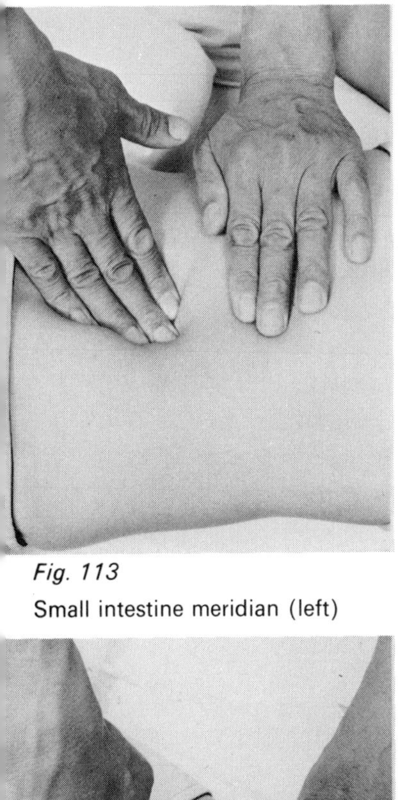

Fig. 111
Kidney meridian (below navel)

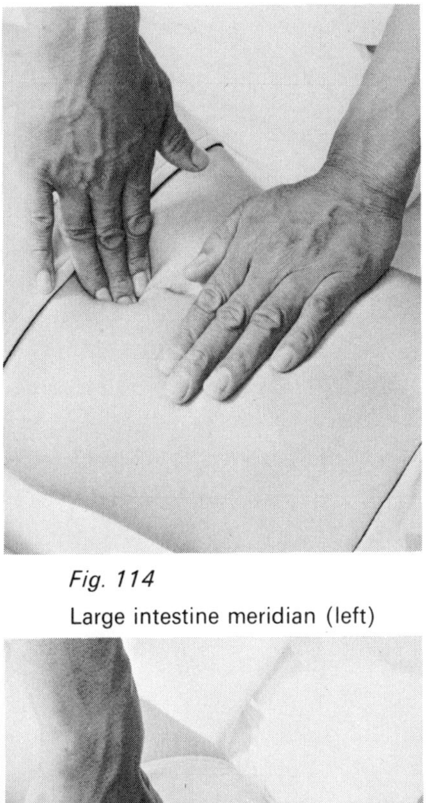

Fig. 112
Bladder meridian (lower hara)

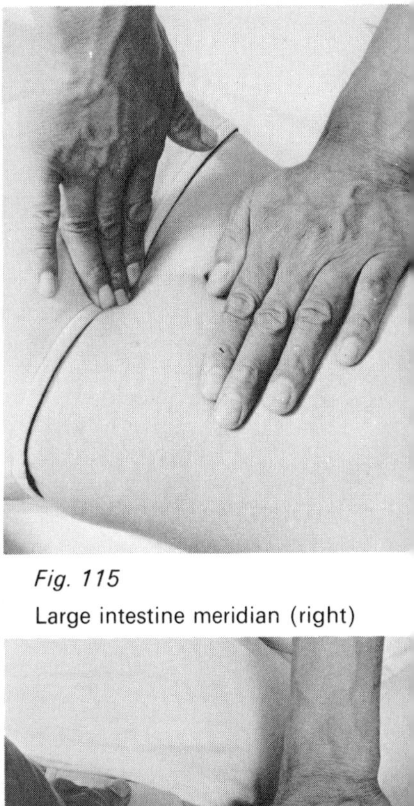

Fig. 113
Small intestine meridian (left)

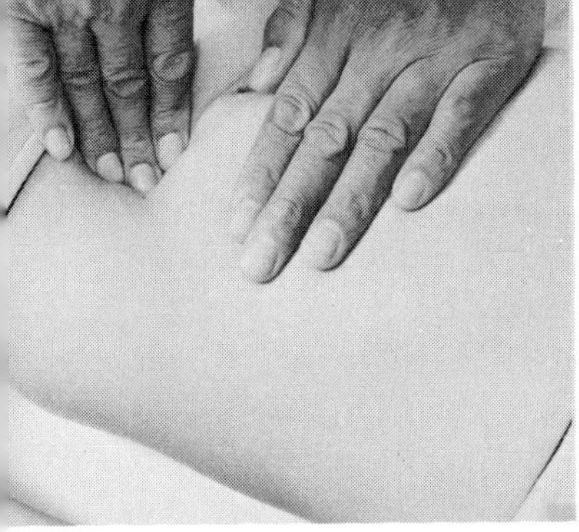

Fig. 114
Large intestine meridian (left)

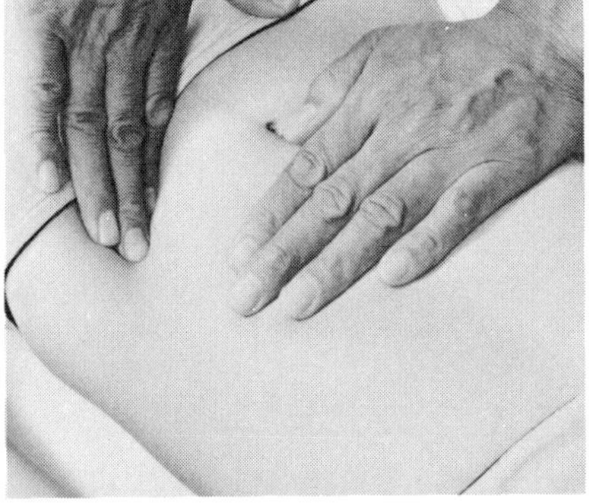

Fig. 115
Large intestine meridian (right)

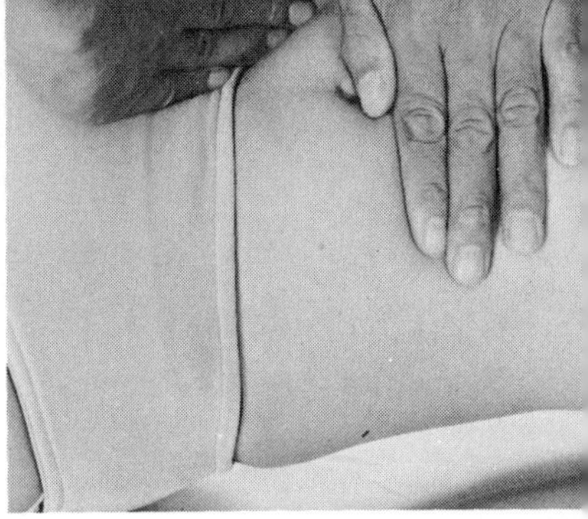

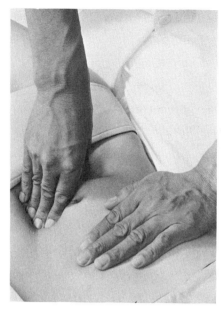

Fig. 116
Small intestine meridian
(both right and left)

Finding Jitsu Points

Hara Diagnosis: After diagnosing the meridians on the hara area, you should find what points are *kyo* and what points *jitsu*. If you are not sure, first place one hand on the supposedly *jitsu* point. Place your other hand on the corresponding point related to the same internal functioning and compare both sides. You should be able to pick up the more *jitsu* side. If you cannot find the *jitsu* point, you may have mistaken a *kyo* point for a *jitsu* point. That is offering resistance or compensating for a *kyo* point located in the same area.

How to Find *Kyo* Point

If you suddenly press hard on the *kyo* area, you will find the area difficult to treat. *Kyo* points usually have a very penetrating stiffness and are very sensitive to violent manipulation. When *kyo* points are "attacked," the entire body will contract in order to defend it.

Muscle Defense

To further explicate the sensitivity of the *kyo* point, let us take a case of appendicitis as an example. If you maintain a steady touch on the hara area, the pain will gradually subside. However, if you suddenly alter the nature of this touch in any way severe pain will result. Thus we can see how important it is to maintain a steady consistent touch when dealing with *kyo* points.

Of course, *kyo* points do not react this way only in the case of acute inflammation like appendicitis. All distortions originate from weak *kyo* points. And just as a weak person becomes more nervous and resistant to a person who is focusing on his weakness, the *kyo* point reacts similarly.

Tonification

Through the process of tonification we can strengthen the *kyo* points and dissipate any stagnation or stiffness in those points. It is important that you approach each *kyo* point gently but firmly. Any sudden or abrupt pressure will cause the point to close up. Slowly manipulate and penetrate the area involved. Then hold and wait until you feel the stiffness subside. Not only the *kyo* point but the patient himself will open up to you resulting in a more effective treatment in an atmosphere of relaxation and trust.

Tonifying the *Kyo* Point

It is very difficult to reach the *kyo* point without any force. It is best that you wait until you feel the point's *Ki* energy coming through. Holding the point, being patient, and waiting for that moment is very important.

Supporting Pressure

Gentle pressure that feels more like support to the patient is necessary in order to find and treat *kyo* points. These points are concealed when the patient is stiff, so relaxation is the key to treating *kyo* points effectively.

Stiffness in the *Jitsu* Points

In conventional shiatsu therapy, one is apt to find the *jitsu* point, which is obvious because the stiffness can be felt, and concentrate on that point. Skilled therapists do not do this. When you find the *jitsu* and corresponding *kyo* point in the *hara*, you hold the *jitsu* point and tonify the *kyo* point. When you tonify the *kyo* point, all the stiffness and resistance in the muscle connected with the *jitsu* point will subside.

Giving Effective Shiatsu

It is very easy, even for beginners, to locate the *jitsu* point because it is on the surface. However, this is not considered oriental medicine. In order to give effective shiatsu, the invisible *kyo* point must be found. This requires practice and increases our knowledge of the real cause of the problem. So the first step is to find the *jitsu* point, confirming the area of stiffness, then tonify the *kyo* point and diagnosis the condition at hand, then check again the area of stiffness. Through tonifying the *kyo* point, you will find that the pain or stiffness is relieved or completely gone.

After completing hara diagnosis, you can give both hands shiatsu on the hara as shown in Fig. 117.

Place the four fingers of both hands on the sides of the hara area. Then place your thumbs beneath the rib cage with your palm resting on

Fig. 117   Fig. 118   Fig. 119

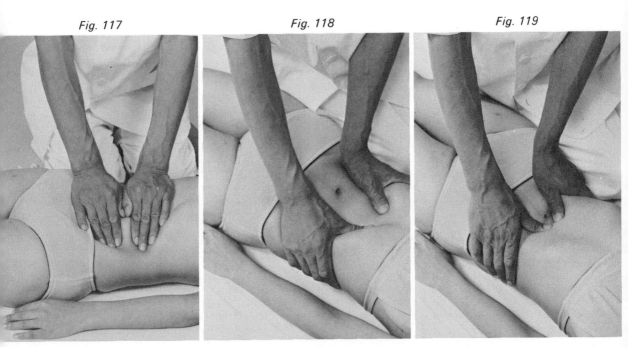

the center of the hara (Fig. 118). As an alternative, you can alternate, first pressing one side and then the next. You will be able to feel the movement inside the stomach and duodenum area. Apply a little more pressure with both thumbs and slide your heels of the palms down to the pubic bone area and hold. Release, then try again. Then slide your thumbs and palms to the groin area along the hara muscles (Fig. 119).

Technique for Leg Manipulation: Diagnosis of the meridian lines in the legs using both hands is useful in confirming *kyo* and *jitsu* in the hara area.

Place your left hand on the lower hara area near the pubic bone and with your right hand apply pressure to the groin area (right and left) (Figs. 120 and 121). Avoid touching the genital area with the fingertips. Without moving your left hand, give palm shiatsu with the right hand from the left groin area to the kneecap (Fig. 121). Do the same to the right groin area. Follow this procedure twice on each side.

Meridian
Stretching
Technique

Expose the inside of the patient's leg by bending it at the knee. Apply gentle pressure to the inside of the thigh and gently squeeze the inside of the lower leg (Fig 123). First you will be able to see the spleen meridian. By bending the leg more acutely, you can feel the small intestine meridian. Bending it still more, you will expose the liver meridian. Give shiatsu to each meridian at least twice. If you find any unbalanced energy in the meridians, give additional shiatsu to that meridian.

Try to bend the leg in the opposite direction so that the outside of the thigh is exposed. Follow the same procedure from the groin to the knee on the outside of the leg (Fig. 124). First you will feel the triple heater meridian. Bending it more, you will feel the gall bladder meridian. Bending it still further is the large intestine meridian. You can change angles by moving the ankle upwards. Bring the patient's knee to her

Fig. 120 *Fig. 121* *Fig. 122*

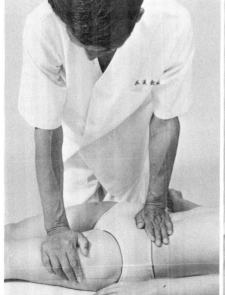
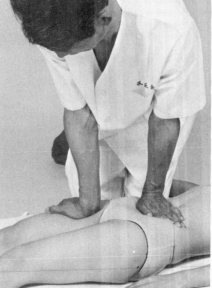
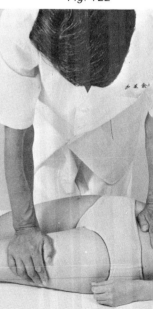

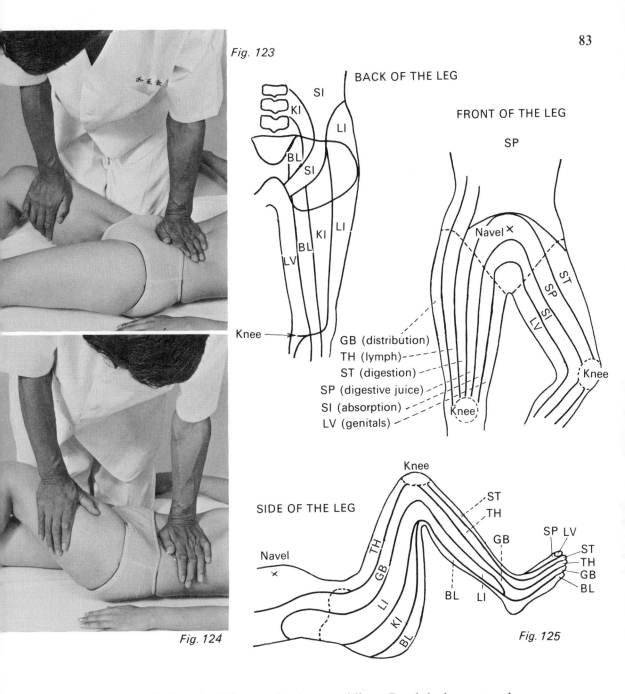

Fig. 123

BACK OF THE LEG

FRONT OF THE LEG

SP

Navel ×

Knee

GB (distribution)
TH (lymph)
ST (digestion)
SP (digestive juice)
SI (absorption)
LV (genitals)

Knee

SIDE OF THE LEG

Knee

ST
TH

GB

SP LV
ST
TH
GB
BL

BL LI

Navel
×

Fig. 124

Fig. 125

chest feeling the kidney and spleen meridians. Bend the leg outward again and you can feel the stomach meridian. Apply shiatsu on the stomach meridian with the right hand.

Do not force the leg outward if the stomach meridian is contracted. Hold her left ankle and place it on her right knee and do shiatsu on the bladder meridian with the thumb and squeeze technique. Repeat a couple of times and feel the *kyo* and *jitsu* points.

One Hand Manipulation
The technique mentioned previously can be done with the left hand remaining on the lower hara while the right hand manipulates and stretches each related meridian lines. Therefore, all these techniques

84

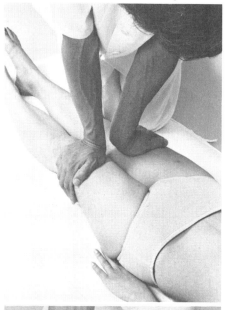

Fig. 126

must be learned with the use of only one hand. Whenever you finish the left side, go on to the right side. You will notice that the stiffness and pain in the hara and leg area will subside and each meridian become less stagnated. The most important part of this technique is the hand resting on the lower hara. This hand must support the patient and play the tonification role. It should also act as a center point for the movement of the legs by the other hand.

After you finish stretching both legs, place both palms on the groin area and with your body weight, apply pressure to the kneecap (Fig. 126). Hold. Then proceed to head shiatsu.

Neck Manipulation: Place a pillow under the patient's head. Then sitting in front of her head, place your four fingers from both hands on the back of the neck on each side with your wrists resting on the pillow. Holding her head gently but firmly, lift her head up stretching the neck area and cervical vertebrae (Fig. 127).

With four fingers supporting the back of the neck, turn her face to the right and with your left thumb, give gentle shiatsu to the left side of the neck (Fig. 128). Turn her head in the opposite direction and repeat the same procedure with the opposite hand (Fig. 129). Remove the pillow and holding her neck and head with both hands, stretch her neck (Fig. 130).

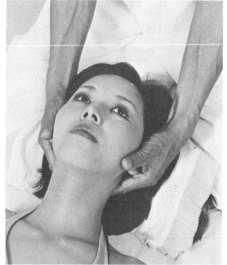

Fig. 127

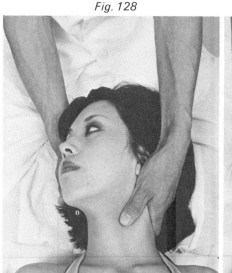

Fig. 128

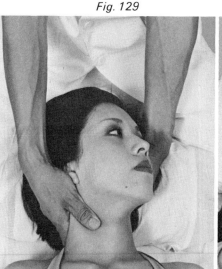

Fig. 129

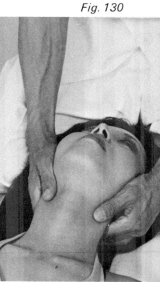

Fig. 130

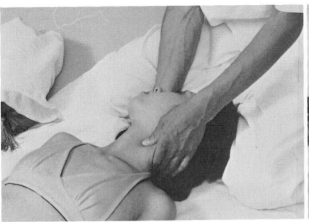

Fig. 131

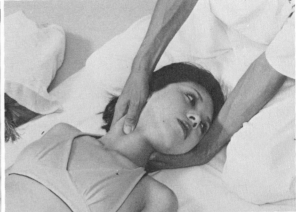

Fig. 132

Turn her head to the right side and give shiatsu gently
to the side of the neck with your thumbs (Fig. 131).
Turn her head to the left side and repeat the same procedure (Fig. 132). Without using a pillow, your thumb can
manipulate deeply because the cervical vertebrae are in a
stretched position.

After you finish warming up your patient's cervical
vertebrae and its muscles, hold the left side of the neck
with your left hand as if you were squeezing it and place
your right hand on the side of her head. Gently turn her
head to the right (Fig. 133). Change hands and repeat
to the opposite side (Fig. 134). Hold the sides of her
head with both hands and turn her head first to the
right and then to the left (Fig. 135). Then straighten. In
this type of manipulation, the supporting hand is more
important than the hand performing the manipulation.

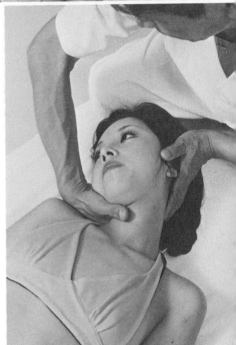

Fig. 133

Fig. 134

Fig. 135

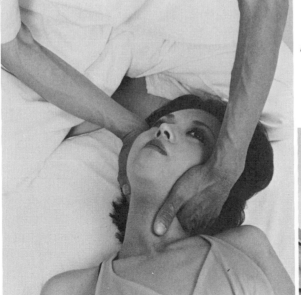

Fig. 136

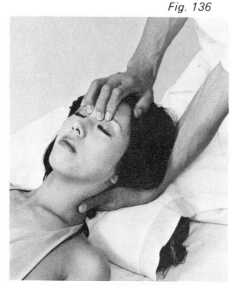

Shiatsu on the Forehead: Place a pillow under the patient's head. Support the back of her head with your left hand and place the four fingers of the right hand on the corner of the eyes. With the palm of the right hand resting on the forehead, lean your body backwards in order to stretch her cervical vertebrae (Fig. 136).

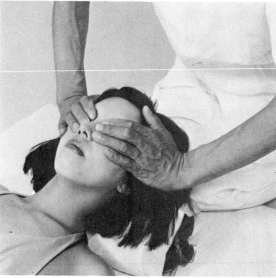

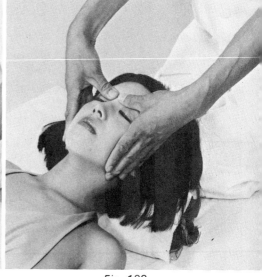

Fig. 137

Fig. 138

Shiatsu on the Face

Place the four fingers of both hands over the patient's eyelids, palms resting on the temples. Hold the position and count to ten (Fig. 137). With the four fingers resting on the sides of the patient's cheek, press the upper eye area very gently (Fig. 138). Then the lower eye area. (Fig. 139). Then the temples (Fig. 140). With the palms resting on the side of the head, place the four fingers of each hand on the sides of the patient's nose (Fig. 141). Give shiatsu to the lower cheekbone area (Fig. 142). Then slide the four fingers of both hands to the jawbone and give shiatsu with your thumbs from below the nostrils to the sides·of the mouth (Fig. 143). Slide your thumb in the direction of your ears from the sides of the mouth to the end of the jawbone (Fig. 144).

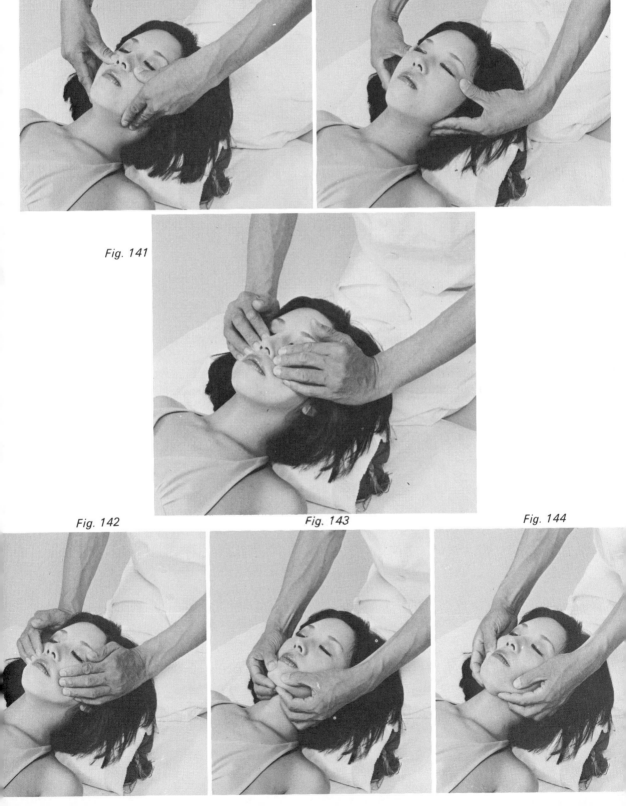

Fig. 139

Fig. 140

Fig. 141

Fig. 142

Fig. 143

Fig. 144

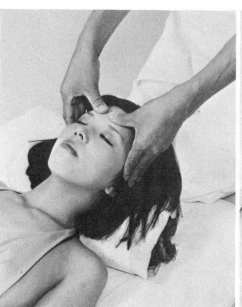
Fig. 145

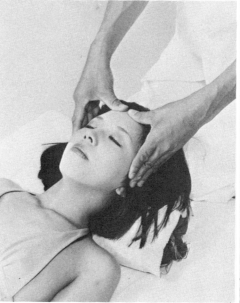
Fig. 146

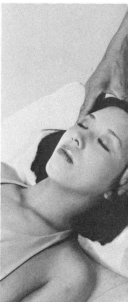
Fig. 147

Do the same as above in the opposite direction. Resting your palms on the sides of her head, place your four fingers of each hand on the temples and hold. Place your thumbs on the center of the forehead and slide toward the temple area (Figs. 145 and 146). You can use three fingers on the eyebrow area. With your thumbs together and your fingers resting on the temples (triple heater meridian area), give shiatsu on the governing vessel (Fig. 147). Then go along the bladder and gall bladder meridians using the same technique from the back of the head to the top of the forehead.

Arm and Leg Manipulation: With the four fingers of each hand resting on the outer chest muscles, place your thumbs on the shoulders (GB-21 area) and hold (Fig. 148). Slide your four fingers down between the ribs to open the rib cage (Fig. 149).

Fig. 148

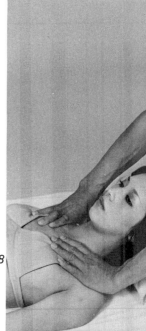

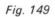

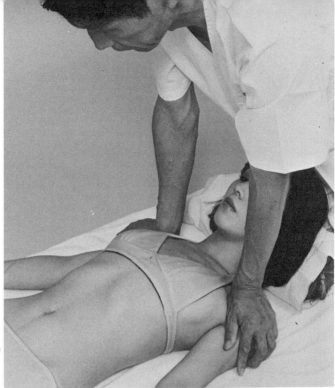

Fig. 150

Fig. 149

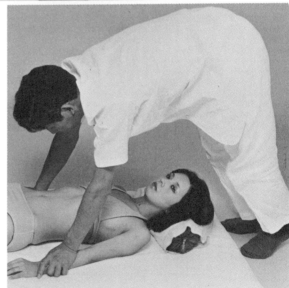

Fig. 151

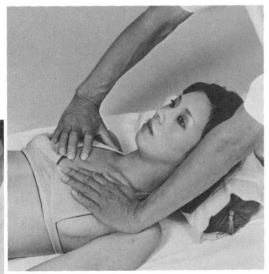

With your palms on her shoulders apply pressure using your body's weight (Fig. 150). This stretches the chest muscles. Gradually slide your palms along her arms, pressing with your body's weight (Fig. 151).

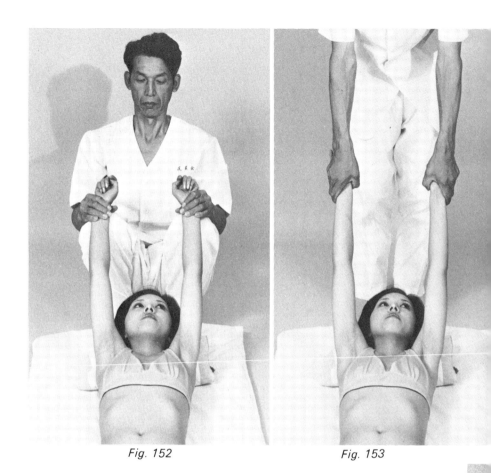

Fig. 152   Fig. 153

Holding her arms at the wrists, raise them toward you. Squat down and place both her wrists on your knees and stretch (Fig. 152). Holding her palms securely, lift her arms again and shake them alternately until they are completely relaxed (Fig. 153). Rotate the arms and place them on the floor with the palms up (Fig. 154). Lift her arms up and to the front crossing them. Pull so that the shoulders are raised a little from the floor (Fig. 155). Let the patient relax. Place both of your arms down to her side and sit down in front of her feet.

Supporting her right foot by grasping the right heel, pull and pinch the toes, starting from the big toe (Fig. 156). Support her foot at the ankle with the four fingers of each hand and press in the arch area using one thumb on the top of the other. Lift her foot a little by grasping the heel with your left hand and give shiatsu with your right palm from the arch to the heels (Fig. 157).

Supporting the patient's right foot with your left knee, stretch her left leg. Rotate her foot, bending the toes back and forth (Fig. 158).

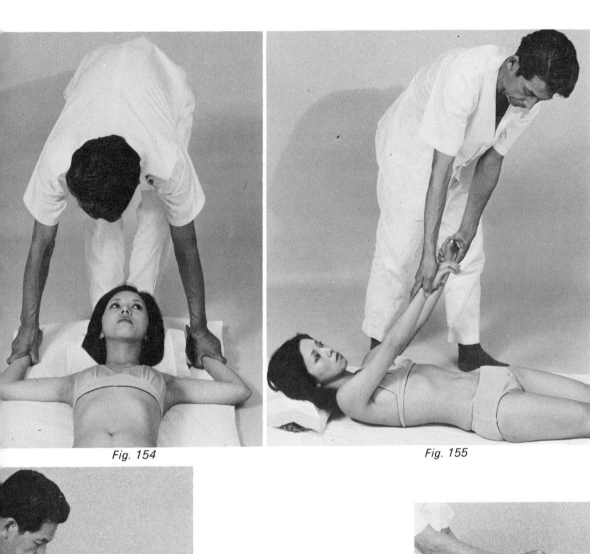

Fig. 154

Fig. 155

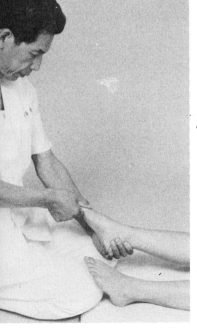

Fig. 156

Fig. 157

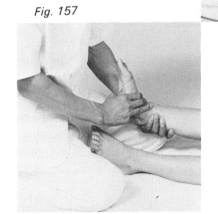

Fig. 158

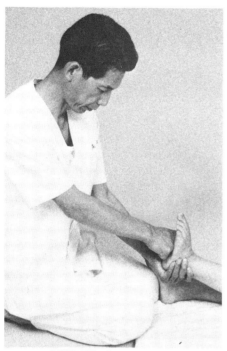

Fig. 159

With your left hand holding the patient's left foot, give shiatsu to the arch using the fist of your right hand (Fig. 159). Repeat to the opposite side.

Stand up and holding her ankles with both hands, place the soles of her feet against your knees. Walk in bending her knees. Support her legs by placing your palms over her kneecaps. Walk in until her knees touch her chest (Fig. 160). If this is not possible, walk in only as far as she can tolerate.

Fig. 160

Fig 161

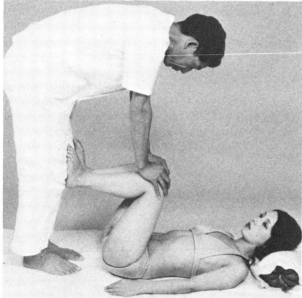

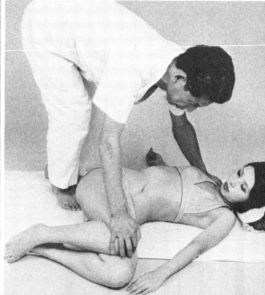

With the patient's legs together and bent at the knees, hold them together at the knees with your right hand. Place your left hand on her right shoulder. Gradually push her legs down to the floor on her left side (Fig. 161). Repeat to the opposite side.

With the patient's legs together, bend her knees again so they touch her chest (Fig. 162). You will find that she will be able to bend her legs more than before. Holding her feet, straighten her legs and shake them several times (Fig. 163). Place her legs straight on the floor.

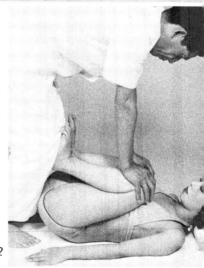

Fig. 162

Fig. 164

Fig. 165

Fig. 166

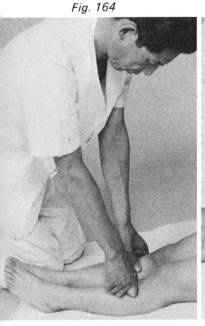

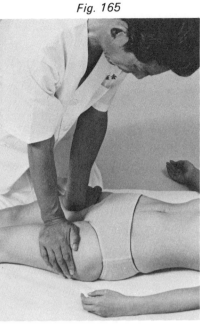

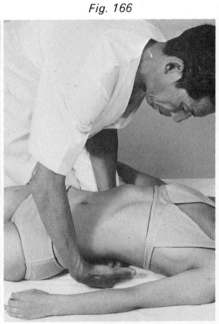

Rechecking the Treated Areas: Give shiatsu along the shinbone with two fingers on each side from the knee to the ankle. You can perform this on both legs simultaneously (Fig. 164).

Rub the area from the ankle to the knee a few times. Change your position so that you are kneeling next to the patient's right knee. Place your palms on both legs near the groin area and give shiatsu down to the knee (Fig. 165).

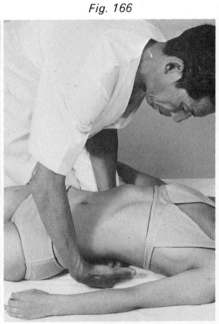

Fig. 163

Fig. 167

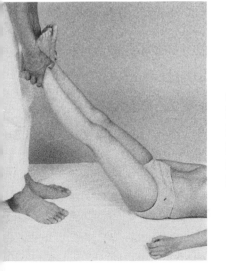

Move your position up to her hips. Supporting the sides of her torso with both palms, gently press on the left and right sides alternately, three or four times. Then hold. Place your fingers on the back of her torso and lift her body slightly and hold (Fig. 166). Gently squeeze the hara area with both hands (Fig. 167) and place the body on floor.

Fig. 168

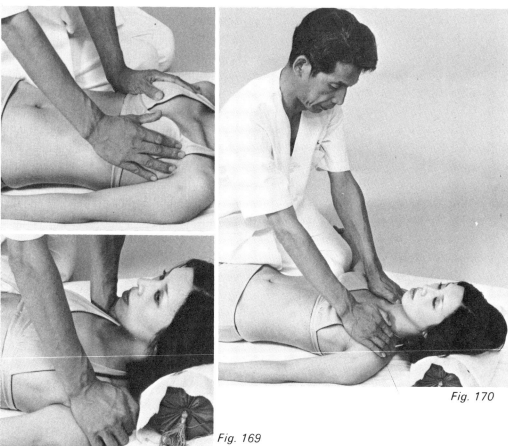

Fig. 170

Fig. 169

Bring your palms to the chest area and gently rotate while pressing (Fig. 168). Do not apply pressure directly on the nipples.

Place your palms on the shoulder joint area and hold (Fig. 169). Grasp both her shoulders and lift them toward you (Fig. 170). Bring your palms to the chest area and quiet her breathing. Cover her with a blanket or towel and remain at her side advising her to please stay and relax from 10–15 minutes.

Treatment Time: The following are approximate times needed to complete the techniques in each position.
  Sitting Position: 7–8 minutes
  Side Position (both sides combined): 12–13 minutes
  Supine Position: 15 minutes
  Prone Position: 10 minutes
  Final Recheck: 5 minutes
Thus it takes approximately 50 minutes for total body shiatsu (10 minutes more in case of specific problems). Beginners have a tendency to take longer while professionals tend to give shorter treatments.

4. Practical Application

Shiatsu without Using Fingertips

Natural Pressure: At this point, there are many misconceptions concerning shiatsu that I would like to clear up. First, it is not true that effective shiatsu requires strong pressure applied with the thumbs and fingertips. Nor it is true that diseases can be cured by merely pressing certain points on the body. Though these techniques are fundamental to shiatsu and useful for the layman to use in his home, professional Japanese masseurs distinguished themselves from amateurs by perfecting the *kyokute* technique which appeared difficult to execute but in actuality was not very effective. In doing so, they ignored more important and effective techniques. The same can occur with shiatsu. Mastering only one technique does not mean you will achieve effective results. In Shinsai Ota's book, *Ampuku Therapy*, he emphasizes that better results can be achieved by simple, innocent techniques than by using only the fingertips. If you ever have a child walk on your back, you will know what is meant by natural pressure. Children are innocent and do not exert an unnecessary amount of pressure. Therefore, when you use your palm, elbow, or knee, be sure that you use a natural amount of pressure.

How to Use Your Palm: Pressure applied with the palm produces a soft, comfortable sensation in the patient and therefore is a very good technique to employ. Strong pressure can also be applied by using the heel of the palm. Another advantage with this technique is that you can avoid fatigue (Fig. 171). It is ideal for ampuku therapy and dealing with the *jitsu* areas in the legs (Figs. 172 and 173).

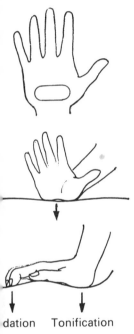

Fig. 171

dation Tonification

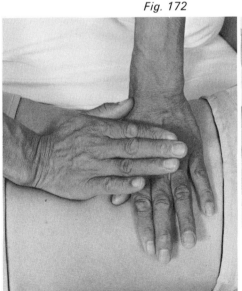

Fig. 172

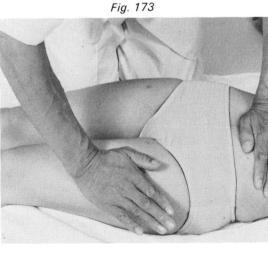

Fig. 173

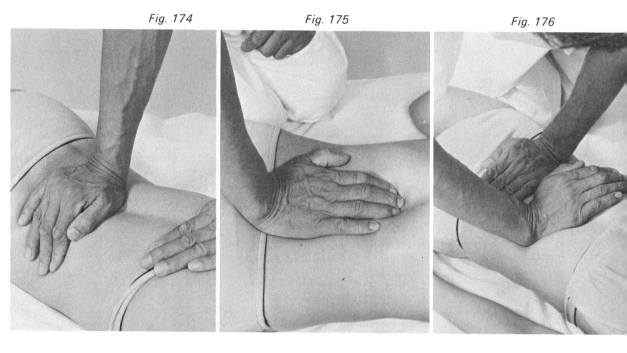

Fig. 174   Fig. 175   Fig. 176

With the patient in prone position, place the center of your palm on the spine. Apply continuous pressure down the spine (Fig. 174). This technique is good for *jitsu* areas because it is not painful. The heels of the palms are better in cases of adjustment and stretching. Remember that pressure should come from your body weight.

You can tonify and sedate with one hand by using your fingers and palm simultaneously. You can press deeply with your fingers while the palm rests comfortably on the surface. Thus you can find the distortion with your fingers and confirm it with your palm. This technique is especially good for ampuku therapy (Fig. 175).

Lean your weight toward the little finger side of your hand to give firm shiatsu. This "knife edge" of the hand is used in karate as a strong destroying technique. However, if it is used softly, it can give deep, effective pressure. This technique is especially good for the area below the rib cage and the groin (Fig. 176).

How to Use Your Fist: When you utilize only one technique, fatigue easily sets in. Therefore, it is important that you balance out one movement by a contrasting one. Tension-relaxation, contractions-expansions, stretching-bending—these are all examples of contrasting movement.

After using your palms, you can give very effective and safe shiatsu using your fists. Most people associate the fist with violence. In the martial arts, the fist is an effective technique for attacking and destroy-ing purposes. However, at the same time, the fists can also be used as a

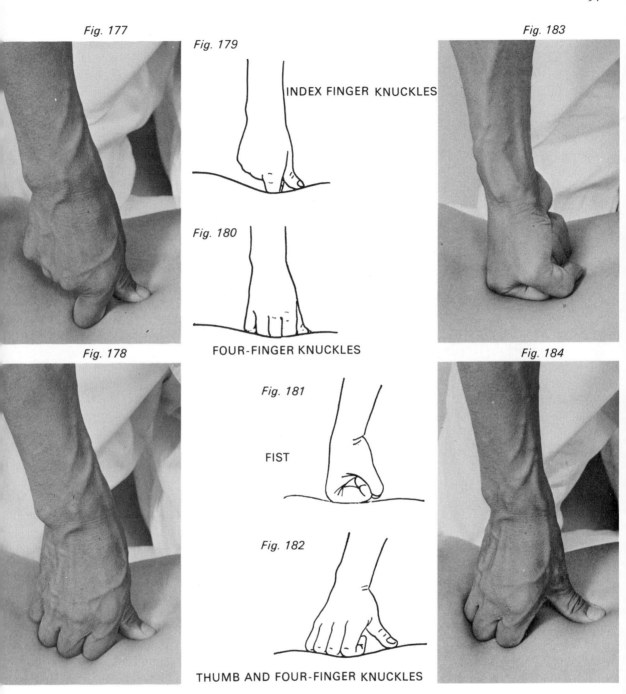

Fig. 177

Fig. 179

INDEX FINGER KNUCKLES

Fig. 180

FOUR-FINGER KNUCKLES

Fig. 183

Fig. 178

Fig. 181

FIST

Fig. 182

THUMB AND FOUR-FINGER KNUCKLES

Fig. 184

technique for revival in cases of unconsciousness. Thus a blow on one point can kill or revive a person depending on his condition. We do not employ such strong techniques in shiatsu. When forming your fists for shiatsu, try not to tense your fingers. Use your body's weight in applying pressure, and you will find that you can give steady, well-balanced shiatsu with your fists without fatigue or damage to your fingers.

How to Use Your Elbow: The elbow is another effective offensive weapon as well as a good shiatsu technique for sedation. However, care must be taken not to apply strong pressure due to the sharpness of the elbow.

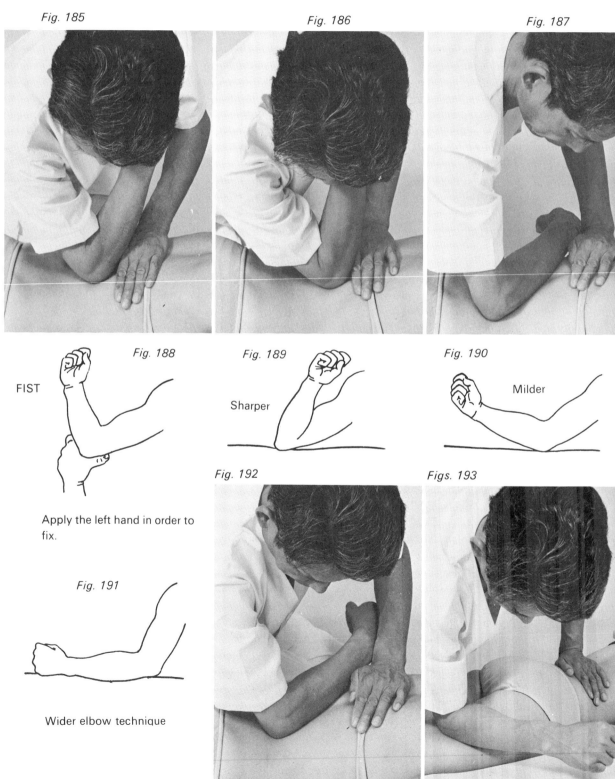

Fig. 185

Fig. 186

Fig. 187

Fig. 188

FIST

Apply the left hand in order to fix.

Fig. 189

Sharper

Fig. 190

Milder

Fig. 191

Wider elbow technique

Fig. 192

Figs. 193

In this technique, rest the elbow on the tsubo and hold it there as if you were resting on your elbow or reclining on your elbow while lying on your side. Do not rotate or force your elbow into the point since this may damage the patient's muscles or joints. If you find it difficult to keep the elbow steady, support it with the other hand.

In Japan, many masseurs develop calluses on their elbows from overuse. This is not natural, nor it is natural to develop calluses on the fingertips.

You can adjust the degree of pressure by changing the angle of the arm. The area between the elbow and wrist can also be used to give pressure to a wider area. Do not under any circumstances use the elbow on the hara area.

How to Use Your Knee: The knee can be a powerful weapon when used in a karate kick; yet it can also be soft and comfortable as a pillow when you rest your head on someone's knee. Knees are bigger and more powerful than the elbows, so be careful using them. It is best to control your body's weight with both hands while pressing with the knee. In this way, you can regulate the amount of pressure being exerted by the knee. Knees are used mainly on the hips, legs, and in cases of stiffness, the arms.

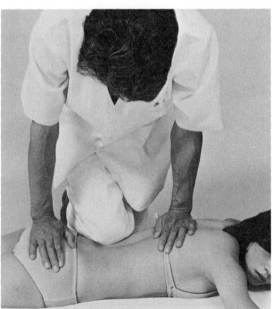 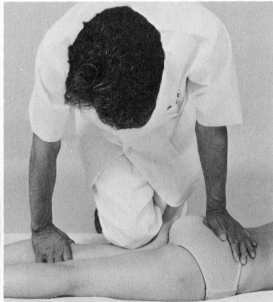

Fig. 194   Fig. 195

Use of Your Feet: If you have ever had a child walk on your back, you can remember how nice that feeling was. You can have an adult do the same thing on your buttocks or legs if they support themselves against a wall, chair, or broom. The movement of walking, whether by the feet or hands, produces a penetrating and comfortable sensation for the patient.

A very effective technique using the feet is to place them on the soles of the patient's feet and apply alternating pressure. This rejuvenates the body because it stimulates an important kidney meridian point (KI-1) that revitalizes *Ki* energy.

Adjusting Technique:　Patients who are abnormally stiff often find that finger pressure alone is not very effective. Some of them boast that they can wear out the practitioner or no matter how hard the practitioner presses, they cannot feel anything. Then there are practitioners who exert excessive pressure to the point of making their patients scream and ruining their fingers. Both ways of thinking are contrary to correct shiatsu philosophy. Excessive pressure only produces more tension and stiffness in the muscle.

If you employ manipulative adjustments to relax the tense muscles, your shiatsu treatment will be much more effective. For example, when our shoulder or arm aches, we instinctively adjust our bodies by stretching the troubled area. In shiatsu, we follow the same instinctive procedure. By stretching the muscle, the patient as well as practitioner, can arrive at a more objective diagnosis of the patient's condition. At the maximum stretch, the muscle has minimum contracting power and offers very little resistance to any pressure applied to that muscle. Thus we can effectively treat this area with less pressure.

In chiropractics, the theory of strong thrusts is employed to correct joint problems. Though this technique pushes the joint back into place, it eventually moves back because the muscles surrounding it have remained in their distorted positions. This can be avoided if you work on the muscles first. With one hand supporting the area at the center point, stretch and rotate the resisting muscle before adjusting. This is a safer and more effective method for treating distortions.

In some chiropractic methods of adjustment, a cracking sound of the bones is indicative of joint correction. This, however, is not a final cure. Without working on the muscles and meridian lines that are connected to our internal organs as well as the joints, lasting results cannot be achieved.

Whole Body Shiatsu

Principle of Sedation

In our fast-paced society, diet and manipulative techniques have taken a secondary role in medicine. In general, diet has been left up to one's "common sense" while manipulation is sought by a privileged few.

Methods of sedation are emphasized in modern medicine because they produce quick results. Therefore, in order to establish themselves with the profession in the same way, manipulative therapy (shiatsu, chiropractics, and osteopathy) must strive for the immediate cure. This is the reason why strong thrusting or strong pressure techniques are considered vogue. The practitioner should be aware, however, of the danger involved in abiding by the principle of the "fast cure." It has been proven that folk medicine, which originally started in the home, has helped in curing chronic diseases and locomotor handicaps that doctors have failed to do because they were looking for an instant cure. Lack of guidance in our medical schools with regard to diet and manipulative techniques is at fault and should be corrected.

When using sedation techniques accurate diagnosis is of utmost importance. This means understanding the existence of *kyo* and *jitsu* in the meridian lines, tonifying, and confirming the degree of distortion taking place within the body. This diagnosis also determines the amount of pressure that should be used with warm-ups. In acupuncture, location of the tsubo is confirmed with the fingertips before the needle is inserted. In this case, you are tonifying as well as confirming. In shiatsu you must check your sedation technique by using tonification techniques that relax the muscles and reduce its resistance.

Sedation Technique—Sitting Position

How to Apply the Elbow to the Back:
After you finish diagnosing the back area, hold the patient's right shoulder with your right hand, and place your left elbow on the left side of the spine around the bladder meridian lines. Turn your left wrist towards her right shoulder. You can place your elbow at a 45 degree angle and lean on your elbow. Slide from the second to eighth thoracic vertebrae and back up again twice. Change and repeat on the opposite side (Fig. 196).

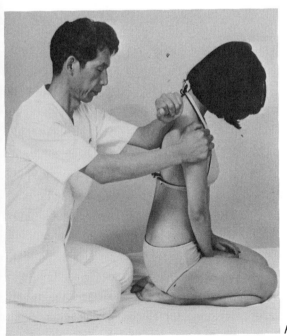

Fig. 196

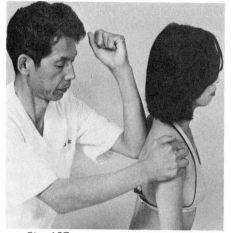

Fig. 197

Do the same as in Fig. 196, applying your left elbow on her left side of the spine from the second to eighth thoracic vertebrae (Fig. 197). Be sure to support your weight on the elbow. Try to bring her shoulder to your elbow instead of pressing the elbow into the shoulder.

How to Stretch the Chest Area: Place your right knee on the second thoracic vertebra area and lean back pulling both her shoulders with you. Repeat with your knee on the area from the fifth to sixth thoracic vertebrae. Do the same for the eighth to ninth thoracic vertebrae area, pulling her shoulder back each time (Fig. 198).

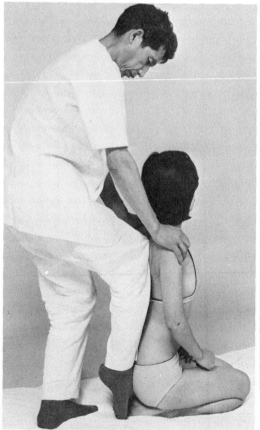

Fig. 198

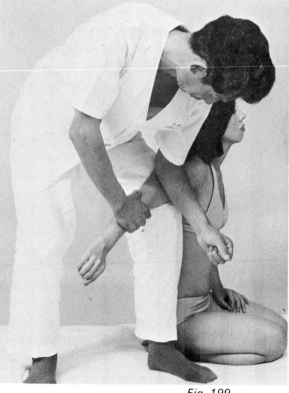

Fig. 199

Using the Elbow on the Arm: After giving general shiatsu on the arms, hold her right elbow with your right hand. Place her upper arm on your left knee and supporting her arm at the elbow, lean on her upper arm with your elbows (Fig. 199).

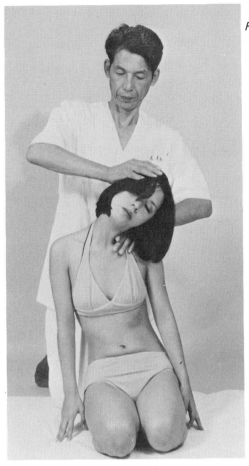

Fig. 200

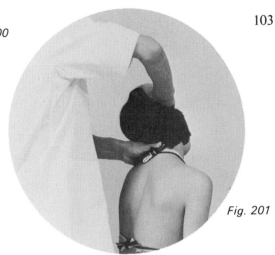

Fig. 201

Fig. 202

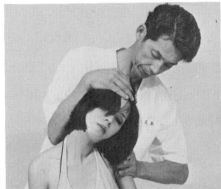

Manipulation of the Cervical Vertebrae: Place the inside of your left thumb on the back of the neck and your index finger on the side of the neck, with the other three fingers resting on the shoulder. Place the right hand on the right side of her head and stretch her neck sideways (Figs. 200 and 201). Place your knee against her back to maintain her erect position while you apply pressure (Fig. 202). You can adjust the degree of pressure by changing the angle of the elbow. A great amount of pressure can be applied using this technique.

How to Stretch the Spine and Cervical Vertebrae

Fig. 203

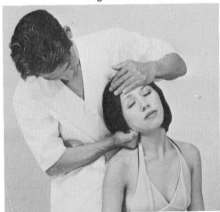

Stretching the Neck: Place your right fist on the back of her neck and your left hand on her forehead. Bend her head backwards into the fist. You can perform this technique on the left and right side as well as the back (Fig. 203).

Hold her head with both hands and lift her head up (Fig. 204).

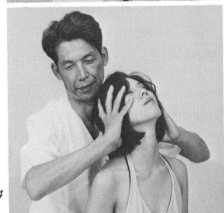

Fig. 204

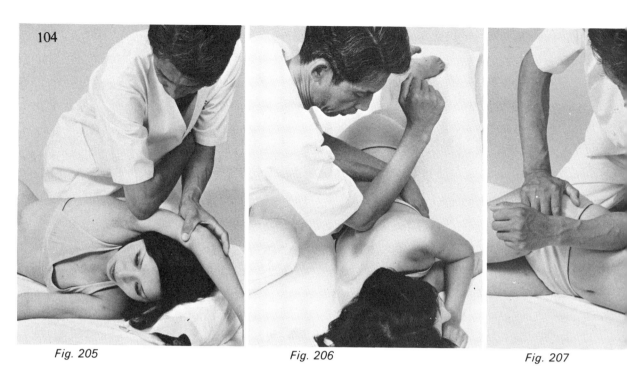

Fig. 205 Fig. 206 Fig. 207

Sedation Techniques on the Side Position

How to Manipulate the Upper Arm: Hold her elbow with your left hand and support the area of the armpit with your right hand (Fig. 205). Hold it. Then rotate her arm in as wide a circle as possible to get the maximum stretch in each position. When moving her arm over her head, try to touch her arm to her ear. Then give shiatsu with your palm and elbow from the patient's elbow to the armpit.

Shiatsu to the Lower Back Area with the Elbow: Support her body by placing your left palm over the hara (beneath the rib cage), resting your right elbow on the side of the hip. Give shiatsu with your elbow along the area of the erector spinae muscles from the top to the lower back (Fig. 206). You can vary the degree of sharpness of the elbow by altering the angle of the bent arm.

How to Give Shiatsu to the Hips: Supporting her hip with your right hand, give shiatsu along the side of the body (along the gall bladder meridian) with your left elbow (Fig. 207). You can increase the amount of pressure by shifting your weight over the elbow. With your left hand supporting the hip area, give shiatsu with your right elbow around the bladder, kidney, small intestine, large intestine, and gall bladder meridians (Fig. 208).

Elbow Shiatsu to the Side of the Leg: Supporting her hip firmly with one hand, give shiatsu along the side of the leg using the elbow or lower arm area (Fig. 209). Begin from the sciatic nerve area down the knee. If

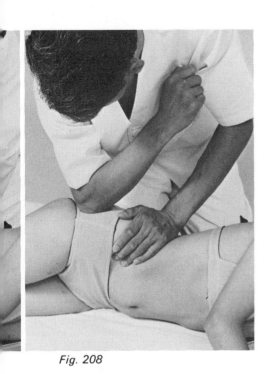

Fig. 208

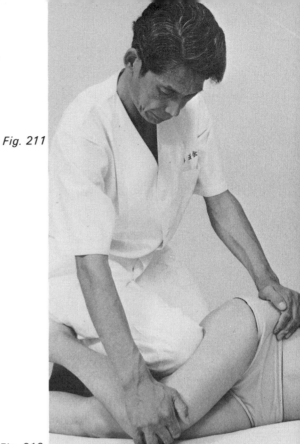

Fig. 211

Fig. 209

Fig. 210

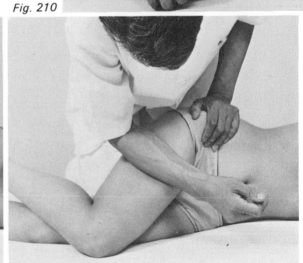

you find a *kyo* point in a meridian line, hold your elbow there for a while and allow it to penetrate the point. You can do the same using your lower arm area instead of the elbow (Fig. 210).

Shiatsu to the Back of the Leg Using the Knee: To stabilize the patient's side position, place one hand on the hipbone and the other on the knee (Fig. 211). Place your knee in back of the leg which is bent in front and pull the patient's leg against the knee (Fig. 211).

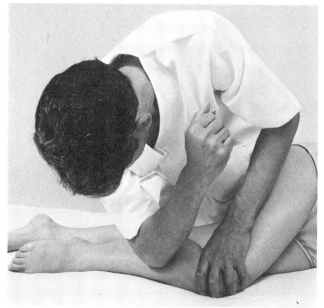

Fig. 212

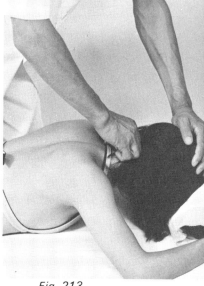

Fig. 213

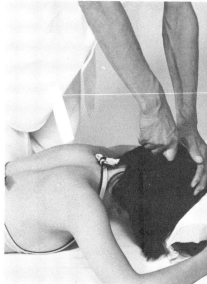

Fig. 214

Shiatsu to the Lower Leg Using the Elbow: Supporting the leg at the knee with one hand, give shiatsu
with the elbow of your other hand down the side and
back of the lower leg (Fig. 212). Repeat on the other
side.

Sedation Technique in the Prone Position

As I mentioned previously, you may rest the patient's
forehead on a pillow when she is lying in the prone or
supine positions, or remove it so that the patient can
lie flat with her head lying to the side most comfortable.

Palm Shiatsu on the Head: Have the patient hold the
pillow under her forehead with both hands. With one
hand supporting her head, press her whole head with
the other hand's heel of the palm or palm (Fig. 213).
Hold each movement before going on to the next.

Stabilize her head by holding the top of her head
with your left hand. Give two-finger shiatsu (bent
index finger supported by the middle finger) from
the top to the bottom of the back of the head (Fig.
214).

Hold her shoulder with one hand and give elbow shiatsu to the base of her head (Fig. 215). You can feel a deep indentation in the area of the ganglia. Then from the top of the cervical vertebrae to the end of the shoulder, give shiatsu 3–4 minutes (Fig. 216). Repeat a couple of times and do on the opposite side.

How to Give Fist Shiatsu along the Spine: Remove the pillow and feel her spine by sliding your hand along the spinous processes. Then place your fist on her spine and lean your weight over your arm exerting pressure on the spine (Figs. 217 and 218).

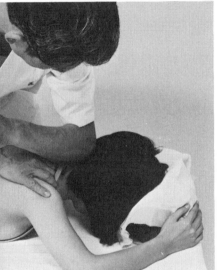

Fig. 215

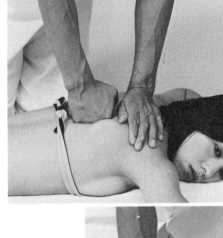

Fig. 217

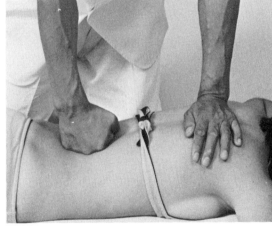

Fig. 218

Fig. 216

Be sure that your position remains stable. You can vary the amount of pressure by applying the fist vertically or horizontally on the patient's back. Try to keep the supporting hand close to the fist to enable your fist to slide along the spine.

Shiatsu to the Back Using the Elbow: You can support your body weight with one hand and give elbow shiatsu to the erector spinae muscles (on the side of the spine) from the first thoracic vertebra to the twelfth lumbar vertebra area (Figs. 219 and 220). Do one side at a time, alternating the pressure from the hand to the elbow and vice versa. There are about 10 major points in this area. This area is very sensitive to sharp pressure, so be careful that you do not "jab" your patient with your elbow. Remember that the weight of your body is the source of pressure coming from your elbow.

The proper feeling for using the elbows should be as if you were lying on the floor with your head propped up on your elbows or sitting at a desk with your head resting on the palm of your hand, elbow on the desk. Avoid using a sharp elbow tip. Many masseurs in Japan develop calluses on their elbows from treating cases of stiffness. This occurs through improper use of the elbows. In dealing with stiff areas, place your palm on the stiff (*jitsu*) point and your elbow on the *kyo* point (Fig. 221).

You can give shiatsu on the spine as well as along the sides of the spine with your elbow or lower arm area (Fig. 222). The palm of the other hand should always be supporting the patient's body in the area being treated by your elbow. After this, you can rub down the patient's back with your palm.

Elbow Shiatsu on the Hips: Place your elbow on the side of the waist pointing in toward the spine. Be careful not to press on the eleventh and twelfth ribs which do not connect fully to the front and do not press on the lumbar vertebrae. Work along the two lines ①② on both sides as shown in Fig. 223. Repeat two or three times (Fig. 224).

Fig. 219   Fig. 220   Fig. 221

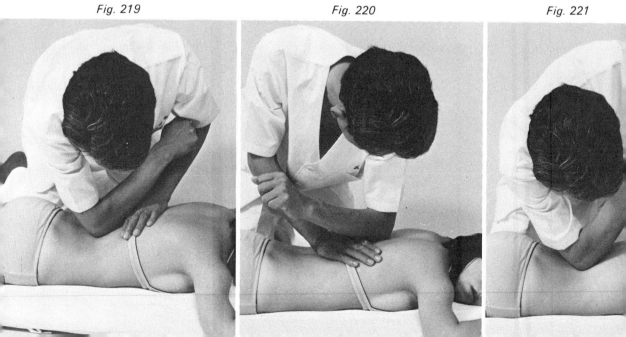

Then from the side of the fifth lumbar vertebra line (③ in Fig. 223) give shiatsu with your elbow down and around the edge of the ilium. Do not press the sacrum with your elbow. Repeat 2–3 times on each side (Fig. 225). Hold your elbow on the hipbone and push down on the patient's body using your own weight. Lastly give palm pressure to the lumbar area by opening up your hands and holding the sides of the patient's waist.

Fig. 224

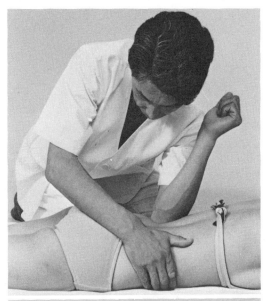

Fig. 223

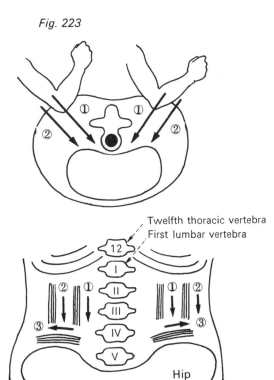

Fig. 222

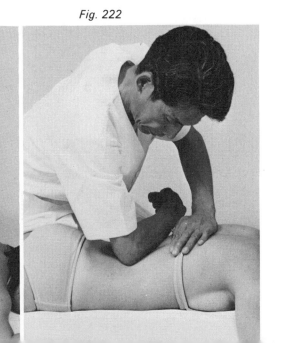

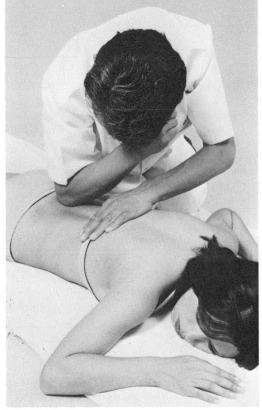

Fig. 225

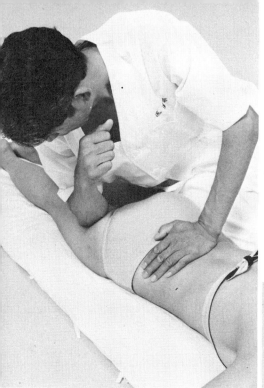

Elbow Shiatsu to the Hips and Back of the Thigh:
With one hand supporting your body weight, give
shiatsu with your elbow to the hip area. Elbow
shiatsu is a good technique to use for this area because of its deep penetration. A sharp elbow tip can
be used in this area (Fig. 226).

Fig. 226

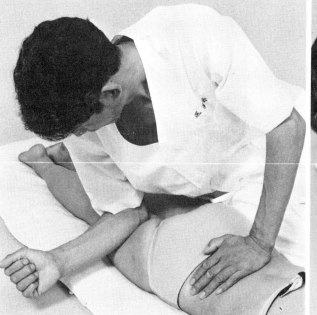

Fig. 227

Keep in mind three imaginary lines—outer, center, inner—going
down the back of the thigh. Give shiatsu with your elbow and lower
arm to the outer and inner lines from the bottom of the buttocks to the
back of the kneecap (Fig. 227).

You can apply more penetrating pressure down the center line with
a sharper elbow.

The other hand should support the patient's body and stabilize the
practitioner's weight at all times (Fig. 228).

Knee Shiatsu   With one hand resting on the buttock and the other on the back of
the kneecap, give shiatsu with your knee. Distribute your weight evenly
on all three points while you hold. You can also give shiatsu to the same
area using both knees (Figs. 229 and 230). Be sure your hands rest on
the hip and knee area.

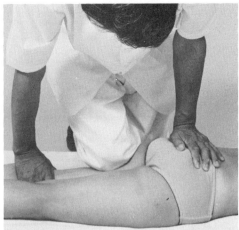

Fig. 229

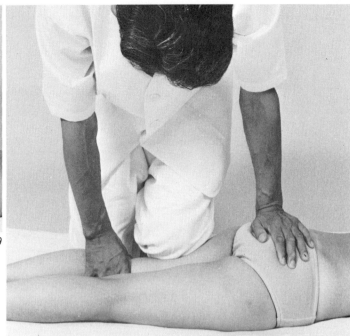

Fig. 230

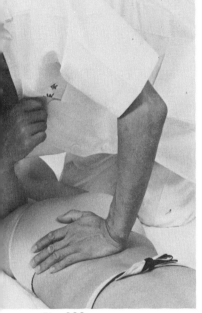

Fig. 228

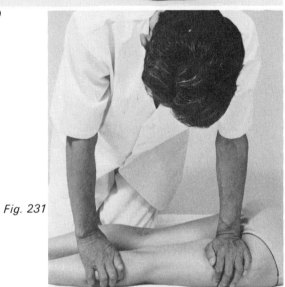

Fig. 231

Give shiatsu with your palms to the
lower leg area from the back of the knee
to the Achilles' tendon (Fig. 231).

Place both of your knees on the arches
of the patient's feet and press using your
body's weight (Fig. 232).

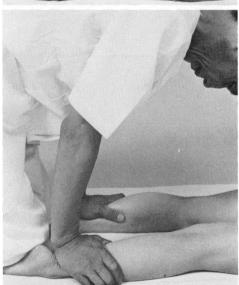

Fig. 232

Standing up, place your heels on the soles of her feet and the ball and toes of your feet on the sides of the Achilles' tendon. Hold. Walk in place on the soles of her feet and hold again (Fig. 233).

Manipulating the Spine: After finishing the back, hold her hip with your left hand and lift up her right leg by the knee and stretch it toward you. Manipulate the spine gently (Fig. 234). Do the same to the opposite side, lifting her left leg at the knee with your right hand and stretching the leg away from you (Fig. 235). In order to prevent the patient's body from twisting, hold her hip area in place with your knee.

Fig. 233

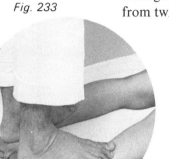

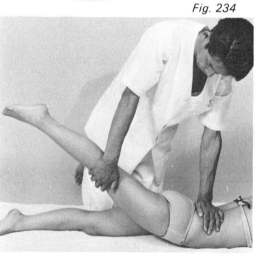

Fig. 234

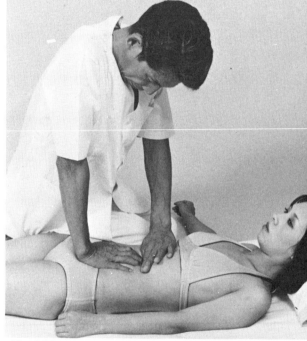

Fig. 236

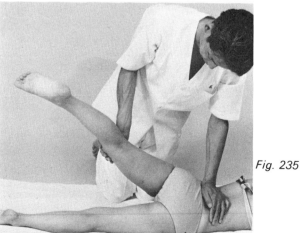

Fig. 235

Fig. 237

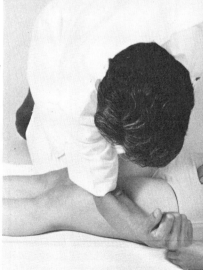

Shiatsu in the Supine Position

Hara Shiatsu Using the Heel of the Palm: When it is difficult to penetrate the hara area with your fingertips, apply pressure using the heel of the palm, thumb, and little finger. Place your other palm nearby to support the hara area with continuous, and even pressure. By doing this, the hara muscles will relax and your palm will penetrate deeper into the tsubos (Fig. 236). Slide your palm to all the diagnostic tsubos mentioned previously. It is important that you apply the pressure gradually keeping the patient comfortable at all times and holding the point for at least 3–5 seconds.

Elbow Shiatsu to the Front of the Thigh: With one hand on the hara giving palm shiatsu, give shiatsu with your elbow to the front of the upper leg (Fig. 237) or with your lower arm (Fig. 238).

You can also use your knee on the front of the thigh instead of your elbow. Because pressure from the knee can be very powerful, be careful not to press hard. To avoid strong pressure, with your knee, place one hand on her knee area and the other on her hara area and balance your body weight between them (Fig. 239).

When moving from one tsubo to the other, transfer your weight from your elbow to the hand resting on the hara and slide your elbow to the next point to the next. Rather, you are transferring your weight from one hand to the other in alternating movements. Be sure that your posture is well-balanced and that your pressure is steady on the patient.

Fig. 238

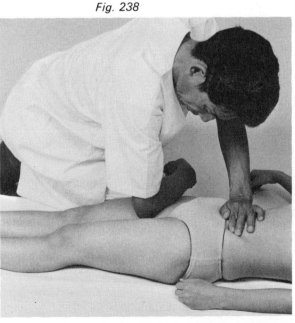

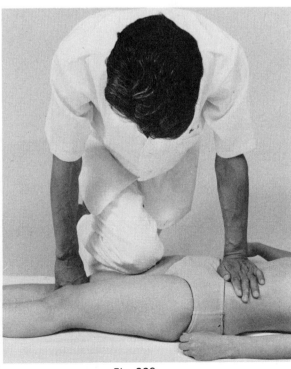

Fig. 239

Fig. 240

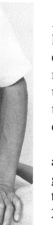
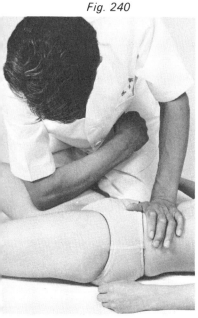

How to Sedate the Legs: The hand that is supporting the hara plays a very important role in the above technique because it calms and reduces muscle tension caused by stress or manipulation in the legs. The effectiveness of manipulation in the legs is reduced by one-half if the hand does not support the hara. It is through this hand on the hara that the general condition of the meridian lines can be felt.

Bend her right leg so that the inside of the foot touches the ankle of her left leg. Supporting the hara with your left hand, give shiatsu along the spleen meridian lines from the groin to the knee using either your right elbow or knee (Figs. 240 and 241). Apply pressure with your elbow or knee, hold, and then transfer your body weight to the left hand that is supporting the patient's hara and slide your elbow or knee to the next point. When using your knee, be sure to support both her hara and the knee.

Move her left leg so that her left foot touches her right knee. With your left hand still on her hara, give shiatsu along the small intestine meridian line with the heel of the palm of your right hand. From the kneecap to the lower legs, hold each point. Move her left foot higher up the leg and give shiatsu along the liver meridian. Bring her left foot still higher up and give shiatsu along the triple heater meridian line toward her knee using your elbow (Fig. 242).

Fig. 241

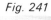
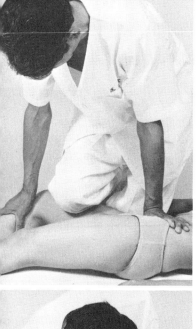

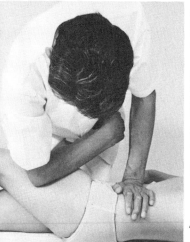

Fig. 242

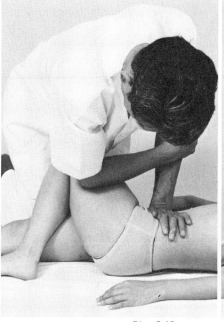

Fig. 243

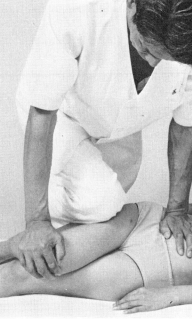

Fig. 244

Rest the patient's left knee on her right knee with her left leg bent outward. Give shiatsu with your elbow along the triple heater meridian. The trick here is to press with your elbow in the direction of her knees as if you were stretching her leg.

Remember that you must be on the same side of the leg you are working on when you are using your knee.

Give shiatsu, using your elbow, along the gall bladder meridian in the same manner as you did the small intestine meridian (Fig. 243). You can use the heel of your palm from the knee to the ankle. You can also use your knee in the same manner as mentioned previously (Fig. 244).

Give shiatsu with your elbow along the large intestine meridian located on the side of the thigh. Push her legs towards the hand that is supporting the hara and then give elbow shiatsu (Fig. 245).

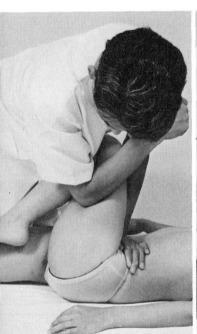

Fig. 245

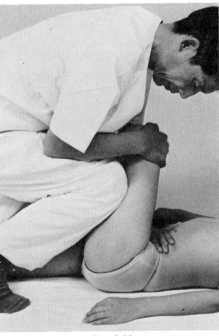

Fig. 246

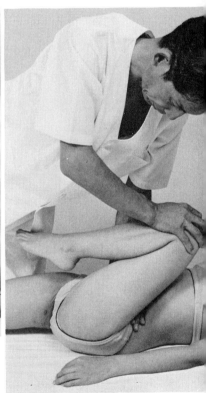

Fig. 247

Supporting her hara with your left hand and knee with your right hand, give knee shiatsu along the large intestine meridian (Fig. 246).

With your left hand still supporting her hara, bring her knee with your right hand up toward the hara (Fig. 247).

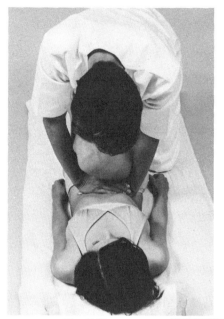

Fig. 248

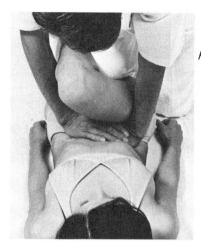

Fig. 249

Fig. 250

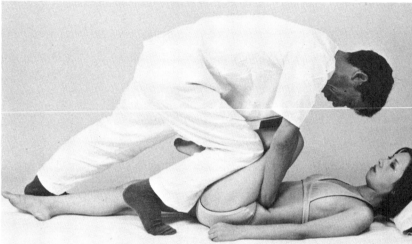

Fig. 251

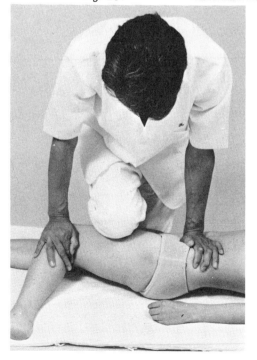

Move your bent knee in the direction of her thigh and place both your hands on the hara (Fig. 248).

Lean forward on her knee so that her thigh presses your hands into the hara (Fig. 249).

In the same position, give shiatsu along the kidney and bladder meridians moving your knee up the back of the thigh to the back of the knee (Fig. 250).

With your left hand still supporting her hara, bend the patient's leg outward so that her knees touch. Give shiatsu with your knee along the stomach meridian (Fig. 251).

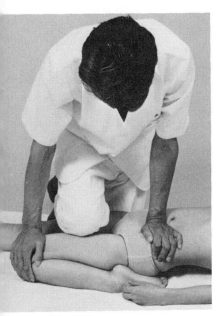

Fig. 252

If possible, hold her toes and bend her leg more in the same direction and give knee shiatsu as seen in Fig. 252. If the stretch involved with this position hurts the patient, stop.

Bring her bent leg towards the thigh of her opposite leg and give thumb shiatsu from the groin to the knee along the bladder meridian. When pressing with your thumb, you can squeeze the other side of the leg with your four fingers.

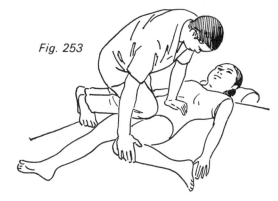

Fig. 253

How to Adjust Subluxations of the Spine: Conventional concepts for treating subluxation problems such as lumbago involve placing the hand on the subluxated area and thrusting it back into place or, as is the case in physical therapy and hospitals, putting the patient in traction. Both of these concepts can make the condition worse and prolong the problem if not done correctly. This makes it difficult for the body to heal itself.

The method I use for correcting subluxations in the area from the tenth thoracic vertebra to the lumbar vertebrae area is simple and very effective.

First of all, it is very important that you understand meridian muscle and organ diagnosis and their location on the back and the hara area. I have explained these locations briefly in Fig. 254, but you can refer to the meridian shiatsu diagnosis chart for further details.

Fig. 254

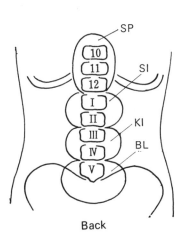

Back

Fig. 255   HOW TO CORRECT SUBLUXATION

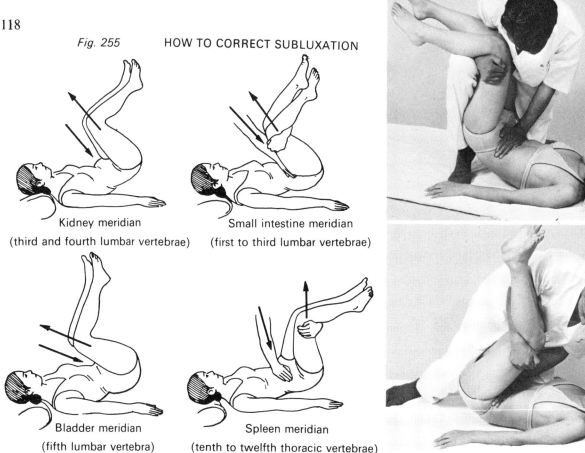

Kidney meridian
(third and fourth lumbar vertebrae)

Small intestine meridian
(first to third lumbar vertebrae)

Bladder meridian
(fifth lumbar vertebra)

Spleen meridian
(tenth to twelfth thoracic vertebrae)

Have the patient lie on her back, rest your left palm on the hara area corresponding to the subluxated area on the back. Place your right arm under her knees, bend them and lift them up (Fig. 256). If you cannot find the subluxated area, you can still follow this general procedure and fix the subluxation indirectly. If this technique is performed correctly, chronic lower backache can be cured in one treatment. However, you should remember that in cases of chronic lower backache, the muscles, meridians, and related internal organs and their functioning are still distorted in the back and hara area so that the subluxation may occur again. So therefore, a total cure may involve many treatments.

Subluxations occurring in the tenth to twelfth thoracic vertebrae corresponding to the spleen meridian is located in the navel area of the hara. With your left hand on the navel, bend her legs with your right arm under her knees and lift her knees up so that the hips leave the floor. Apply pressure to the hara at a 90 degree angle. Because the patient's knees will come close to your face, be sure your body is steady. If you try to thrust, the patient will contract her muscles making this method ineffective. So therefore, when the patient's hips leave the floor, place her bent legs on your right knee and support them with your right elbow and hold. You can stabilize her body by placing your lower right leg against her hips. In this position you can feel with your left hand the patient's muscles relax.

Fig. 256

If you want to achieve better results, you can sink your left hand further into the hara in the direction of the subluxation while lifting her legs up further. Be careful not to push down suddenly. Be cautious using this technique until you are well-acquainted with this method. It is less dangerous than the traditional chiropractic method and can be employed without the use of an adjustment table.

If you spread your thumb and little finger outward in the form of the letter A you can apply even pressure with both hands and their four fingers or the four fingers and heels of the palms. You can further manipulate by lifting the legs, as mentioned previously, and bending them deeper into the hara area.

In the first to third lumbar vertebrae area, related to the small intestine meridian, subluxations can occur laterally as well as vertically. In the case of lateral subluxations, you can place your hand supporting the hara to either side and use the patient's thigh to press the hand into the hara (Fig. 257). Be sure that you press at a 90 degree angle into the hara and that you do not squeeze or twist the hara area.

Fig. 257

The area between the third to fourth lumbar vertebrae is related to the kidney meridian. People who have a weak tanden (lower abdomen) have a tendency to subluxate in this area. It is unfortunate that modern education places too much emphasis on the brain and neglects the tanden because the lower area of the stomach is nature's real source of strength. A weak tanden can also lead to slipped discs and hernia. Using this technique in this area not only corrects subluxations but also aids in building up the tanden, so employ this technique frequently. The procedure is the same as for small intestine meridian for lateral as well as vertical subluxations.

The fourth to fifth lumbar vertebrae is related to the bladder meridian. Pressure should be applied close to the pubic bone. When the patient relaxes and offers no resistance in the hara, you can penetrate the hara area deeply with your hand.

Fig. 258

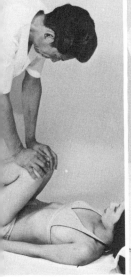
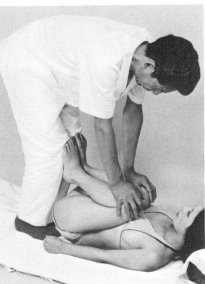

Stretching the Spine: After correcting any subluxations, bring her knees to her chest (Fig. 258). Press her knees down to her chest as far as possible (Fig. 259). This technique is very good to use following correction of any spleen meridian (the tenth to twelfth thoracic vertebrae) subluxations.

Fig. 259

Fig. 260

Fig. 261

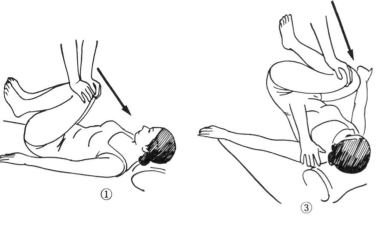

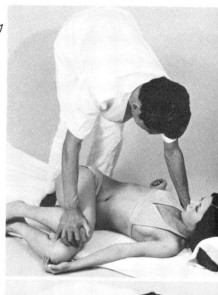

①

③

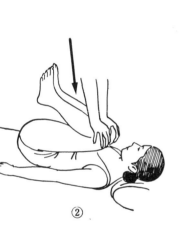

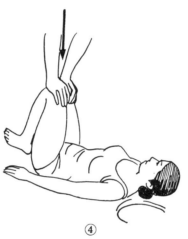

②

④

Fig. 262

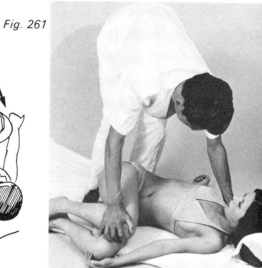

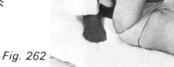

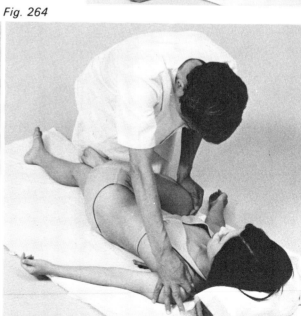

Fig. 263

Fig. 264

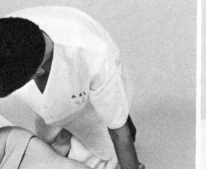

After pressing her knees, place one hand on her shoulder and twist the legs to the opposite side (Fig. 261). The technique is good for reconfirming corrections of any subluxations.

Bring her knees back and place her legs bent on the floor at a 60 degree angle to the body. Push down on both knees toward the coccyx. Keeping the legs in this position, you can turn them to the left or right side to reconfirm lumbar adjustments (Fig. 262).

Bend one leg at a 90 degree angle and push it to the opposite side. Repeat to the other side. This is a very effective stretch when the gall bladder meridian is *jitsu* (Figs. 263 and 264). Bring her knees to her chest once more as in Fig. 258 and you will find that her stretch will have increased.

Shiatsu to the Arms Using the Knee: With the patient lying on her back, stretch both arms out to the side. If there is a gap between her arm and the floor, place a cushion under the gap. Place one hand on her shoulder and the other at her elbow. Give shiatsu with one or both

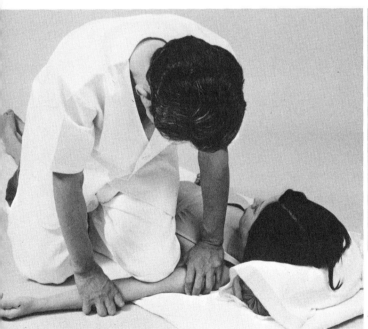

Fig. 265

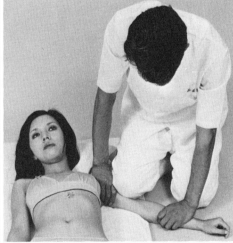

Fig. 266

knees to the distorted meridians. You can give knee shiatsu to her lower arm by supporting her elbow and wrist (Figs. 265 and 266).

These manipulative techniques will improve the results from the general shiatsu procedures. Do not exert strong pressure until you are skilled in executing these techniques. It is also good to remember the benefits of incorporating the maximum stretch principle into your shiatsu treatment.

Exercises of the Meridians

In doing these exercise, do not bounce in position. At the maximum stretch point, stay there and take two deep breaths and try to feel the energy flow in the meridian lines involved. The more you relax, the further you will be able to stretch. The purpose of these exercises is not to develop the muscles but rather as a way of diagnosing the condition of the meridians. Any abnormality or malfunctioning of the meridians can be detected in this way and then corrected to prevent fatigue and sickness. It is important that you keep your body as flexible as possible, and these exercises will aid you in achieving a balanced and supple body.

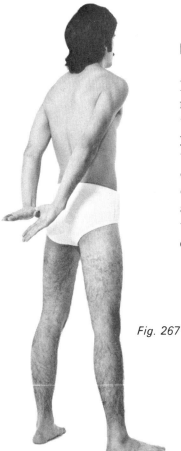

Fig. 267

Fig. 268

(1) *Lung and Large Intestine Meridians*
Cross your hands behind your back (Fig. 267). Bend forward and lift your arms as high as possible (Fig. 268). This exercise stretches the lung and large intestine meridians.

(2) *Stomach and Spleen Meridians*
Sit down with Japanese style and cross your hands. Stretch them as high as possible over your head (Fig. 269). Bend straight backwards from that position until your back lies flat on the floor (Fig. 270). Hold for two breaths. This exercise promotes a healthy energy flow. If you need to stretch more, do the above with your palms turned up toward the ceiling. This exercise stretches the stomach and spleen meridians.

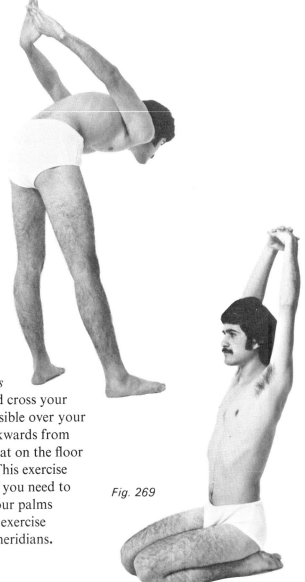

Fig. 269

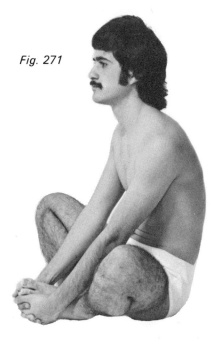

Fig. 271

(3) *Heart and Small Intestine Meridians*

With the soles of the feet together, bring your feet towards your body as close as possible (Fig. 271). Holding your feet with your hands, try to touch your head to your toes, resting your elbows on the foor (Fig. 272). Relax completely and take two deep breaths. If your knees do not lie flat on the floor, this indicates malfunctioning of the heart and small intestine meridians. If one side is higher than the other, a problem may exist in those meridian lines on that particular side. This exercise stretches the heart and small intestine meridians.

Fig. 272

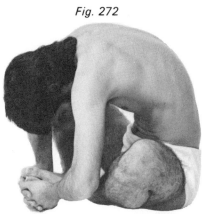

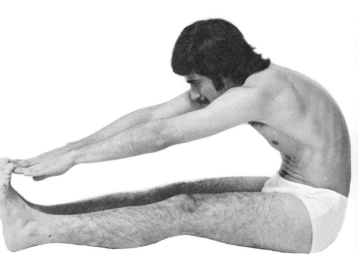

Fig. 273

(4) *Kidney and Bladder Meridians*

Stretch your legs straight out in front of you and touch your toes with your hands (Fig. 273). Then bend forward and touch your head to your knees. At the maximum stretch point, relax completely and take two deep breaths. Any pain you may feel on one side indicates malfunctioning of the meridians on that side. This exercise stretches the kidney and bladder meridians.

Fig. 270

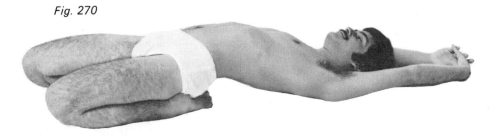

124

Fig. 274

(5) *Heart Constrictor and Triple Heater Meridians*

Sit in the lotus position or half lotus position if possible. Cross your arms and hold the opposite knees (Fig. 274). Bend forward and rest your head on the floor (Fig. 275). Hold and take two deep breaths, relaxing completely. Stiffness in the arm indicates malfunctioning of the meridians. This exercise stretches the heart constrictor and triple heater meridians. Under complete relaxation, you can sense any distortions in the meridians much more clearly.

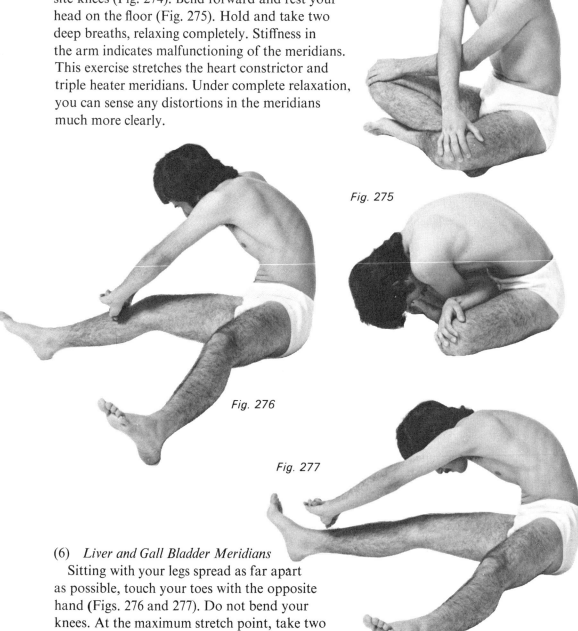

Fig. 275

Fig. 276

Fig. 277

(6) *Liver and Gall Bladder Meridians*

Sitting with your legs spread as far apart as possible, touch your toes with the opposite hand (Figs. 276 and 277). Do not bend your knees. At the maximum stretch point, take two deep breaths and relax completely. Any stiffness you may feel indicates malfunctioning of the meridians involved. This exercise stretches the liver and gall bladder meridians.

5. Self-shiatsu

Though the basic purpose of shiatsu is to give and take with another person, there will be times when you will not be able to do this. When you have no other alternative, practice self-shiatsu. The Zen monk, Hakuin, fell sick once because of some difficult exercises he did while practicing Zen. He was able, however, to cure his disease through self-diagnosis and self-shiatsu.

The advantage of learning self-shiatsu is that it can be practiced anywhere and anytime without any preparation or instruments. It can be practiced when you are studying, working, waiting for your train or bus, or when you are simply by yourself.

How to Practice Self-shiatsu

The most difficult tendency to overcome when learning self-shiatsu is tensing your fingers when applying pressure to your body. This is not good shiatsu. When you learn to relax your fingers and apply soft pressure, you will find that you will penetrate deeper into your body and feel the meridian lines. This feeling is also important when giving shiatsu to another person.

Fig. 278

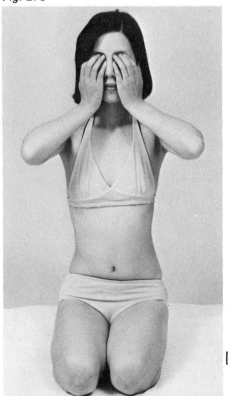

Sitting Position

First rub down your entire face, head and neck as if you were washing them.

Shiatsu for the Eye Area: Cover your eyes with your hands and apply light shiatsu (Fig. 278). The fingers of both hands should be resting on the upper lids and instead of pressing toward your eyes, bring your face to your fingers.

[125]

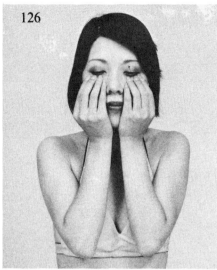

Fig. 279

Place your four fingers on the lower eye area and give shiatsu as if you were pulling your wrist down (Fig. 279).

Place the four fingers of each hand on the temples with your thumbs resting on the sides of the jawbone. Give shiatsu to the temple area (Fig. 280).

Rest the thumb and index finger of your left hand on the sides of your nostrils. With the right thumb and index finger on the left thumb and index finger, press this area (Fig. 281). Repeat two to three times.

Again cover your eyes with your fingers and apply gentle shiatsu by bringing your face to your fingertips (Fig. 282). Hold for 3–5 seconds. You can use these techniques when you are reading a book or studying or resting after a long drive. It is also very good in relieving fatigue or heaviness in the head in a short period of time.

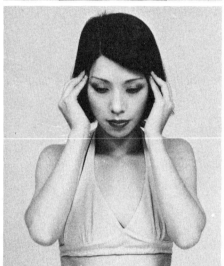

Fig. 280

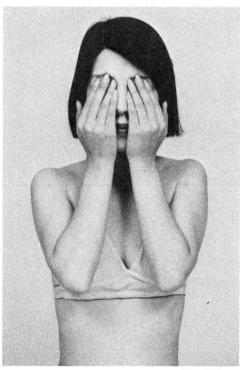

Fig. 282

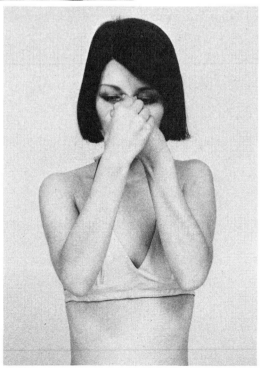

Fig. 281

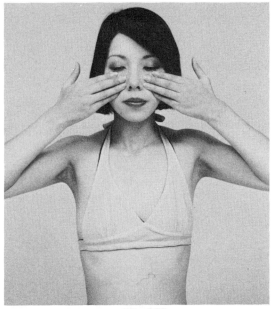

Fig. 283

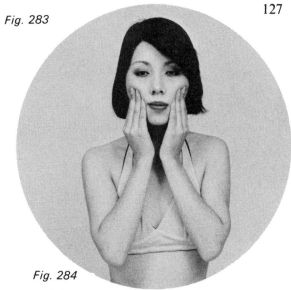

Fig. 284

Fig. 285

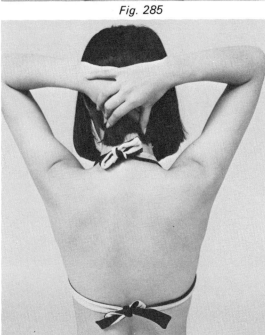

Fig. 286

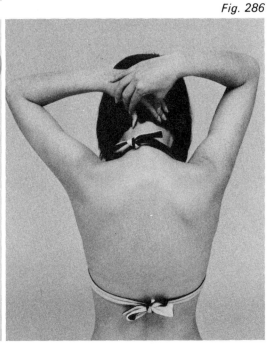

Nose Shiatsu: Shiatsu for the nose is very effective for nasal congestion, running nose, and fever.

Place your fingers on the side of your nose and press inward like you were pinching your nose (Fig. 283). This technique promotes good blood circulation in your mucus membrane. Hold for a while. You can achieve better results by applying hot towels to this area.

Press your cheekbones with both hands (Fig. 284).

Place a hot towel on the back of your neck and press the back of your neck with your thumbs (Figs. 285 and 286).

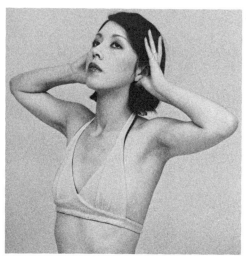

Fig. 287

Move your thumbs to the edge of the skullbone and apply pressure by bending your head backwards (Fig. 287).

Slide your thumbs outward a little further (GB-20 area) and apply pressure the same way as in Fig. 287. This shiatsu is very good for eye problems.

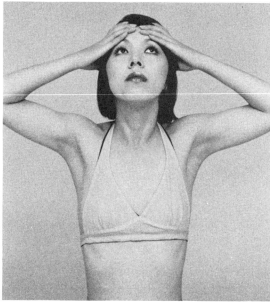

Fig. 288

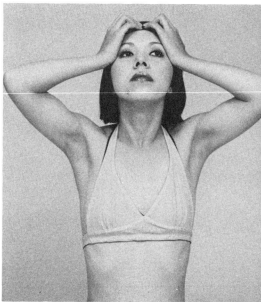

Fig. 289

Place your fingers on your forehead and slide both hands outward while applying light pressure (Fig. 288). With your fingers placed on your forehead place your palms on the side of your head. Gently squeeze your head with your palms and apply pressure with your fingers by pulling your wrists down. Proceed from the forehead to the top of the head and then slide down the back of the head on both sides (Fig. 289). Give shiatsu on the bladder meridian lines from the front of the head to the top of the head (Fig. 290). This technique is very good for headache and sleepiness.

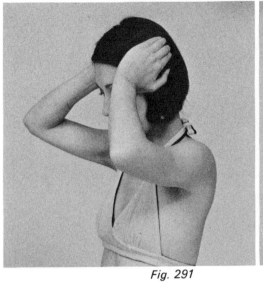

Fig. 291

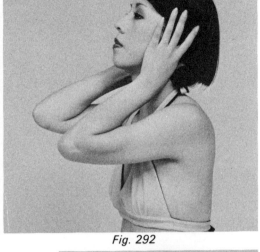

Fig. 292

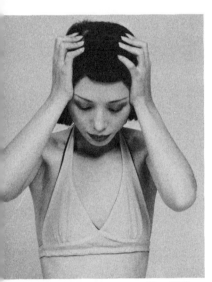

Fig. 290

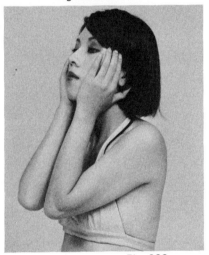

Fig. 293

Head Shiatsu: Place your hands on the sides of your head as if you were covering your ears and give shiatsu to the gall bladder, triple heater meridians, and governing vessel lines (Fig. 291).

Back of the Head

Place your thumbs in the center of the back of your head near the occipital protuberance area and rest your fingers on the sides of your head. Supporting your face with your fingers, press the back of your head with your thumbs from the center to the lower ear. Follow the line of the cranium (Fig. 292).

Sides of the Head

Place your fingers near the temples and give shiatsu with the heel of the palm under the jaw. Slide your palms from the center of the jaw to the bottom of the ears (Fig. 293).

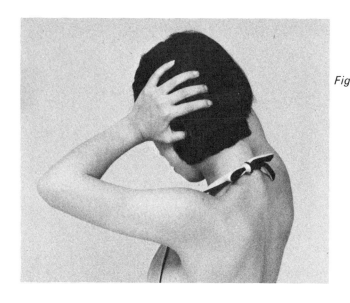

Fig. 294

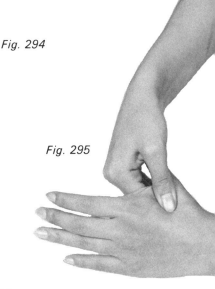

Fig. 295

Back of the Head

With your fingers on the back of your head and the heels of your palms on the side of your head, squeeze your hands against your head (Fig. 294). Release, then move your hands, in the same position, down toward the ear and repeat.

This technique is very effective for concentration, sleepiness and calming your nerves. After completing this, give hand shiatsu.

LI-4

Pinch LI-4 which is located between the thumb and index finger. You can also press the same point (Fig. 295).

Throat Shiatsu: Place both hands on the parotid area near the ear and rub down. Slightly pinch the ear with your index finger and middle finger (Fig. 296).

Shiatsu for Rejuvenation

The hormones secreted by the parotid are essential in staying younger so the tsubos located in this area can be pressed to rejuvenate (Fig. 297). These points are also good for stimulating saliva secretion.

Fig. 296

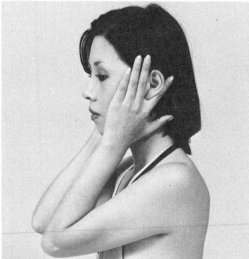

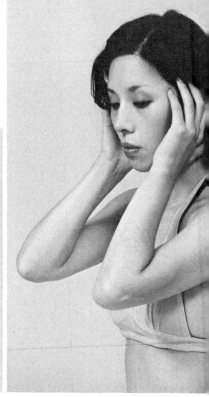

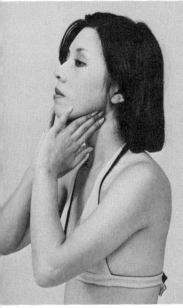
Fig. 298

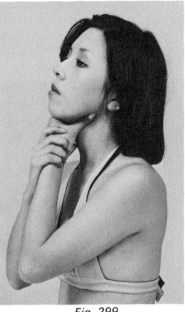
Fig. 299

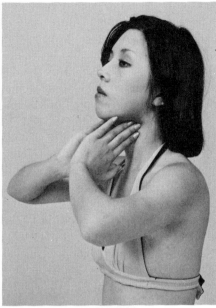
Fig. 300

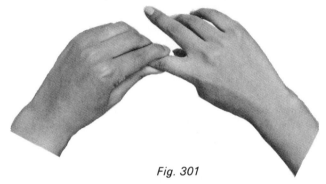
Fig. 301

Fig. 297

Nasal Stagnation

Place your fingertips beneath the jaw and press upwards. If you touch your tonsils and find it painful, give shiatsu very gently until the pain subsides (Fig. 298).

Throat Shiatsu

Place your thumb on one side and the fingers on the other near the parotid area of the neck. Give shiatsu down the neck and thyroid area (Fig. 299). Stiffness will occur in this area when you have throat problems.

Place your four fingers of each hand on both sides of the trachea and gently squeeze (Fig. 300). Press from the jaw to the collarbone.

Large Intestine Meridian Lines

Pinch your index finger with two fingers of the other hand (Fig. 301).

You can perform the techniques for face, head, and neck with one hand if it is impossible to use both hands. In all cases, make sure that you apply soft pressure. When one hand is occupied with doing something else, you can give shiatsu to yourself with the hand that is free. In this case, use your thumb, four fingers, and heel of the palm all together in order to give steady, continuous pressure.

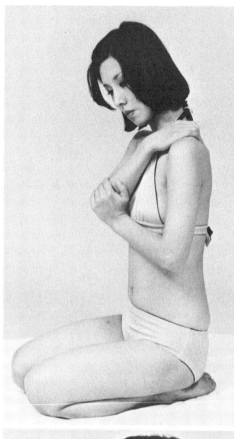

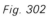
Fig. 302

How to Give Shiatsu to the Shoulders: Stiff shoulders are so common and indicative of many ailments that shiatsu alone will not be able to cure the main cause for the condition. It is difficult to give shiatsu to one shoulder without tiring the other shoulder, so it is advisable that shiatsu is combined with exercise to help relieve this problem. In cases of pain, self-shiatsu to the shoulders is helpful. Place your hand on the opposite shoulder and give shiatsu while the free hand supports the hand giving the shiatsu at the elbow (Fig. 302). This technique is better than using only one hand without supporting it.

When you are giving shiatsu to one shoulder you can exercise your elbows by moving it with the supporting hand (Fig. 303). You can also move your neck while giving shiatsu to the shoulder. Raising the elbow with your supporting hand helps toward the effectiveness of the treatment (Fig. 304). Give shiatsu to both sides using the maximum stretch.

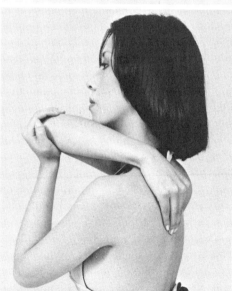

Fig. 303

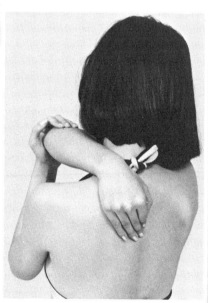

Fig. 304

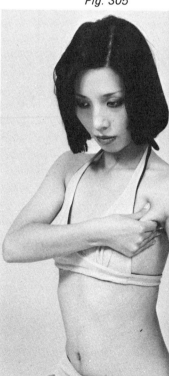

Fig. 305

How to Give Shiatsu to the Upper Arms: If you suffer from shoulder stiffness, you will need shiatsu on the arm too. Stiffness in the arms is also a common problem today.

With your fingers resting on the back of the scapula, press and squeeze your armpit with your thumb (Fig. 305).

Give gentle shiatsu with your thumbs around the shoulder joint (Fig. 306).

How to Stop Toothaches The most important part of the arm is the root of the arm (armpit) and pectoralis major muscle, and the deltoid muscle in the back of the arm.

Treatment of these muscles are good for toothaches. The pectoralis major muscle is good for lower toothaches and the deltoid muscle for upper toothaches. You can also give shiatsu to the arm along the large intestine, heart, lung, heart constrictor, and small intestine meridians.

With your four fingers in your armpit, press the pectoralis major muscle with your thumb and then squeeze it. You may feel a sensation from the front of the neck to the tooth if you are pressing the correct tsubo. Apply as much pressure as desired.

You can squeeze your shoulders from front to the back and give soft shiatsu (Figs. 307 and 308).

Fig. 306

Fig. 307

Fig. 308

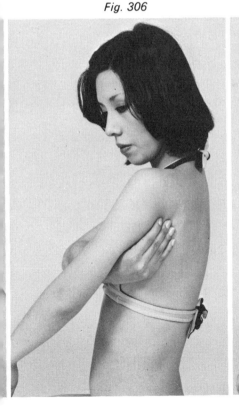
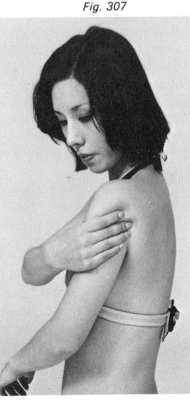
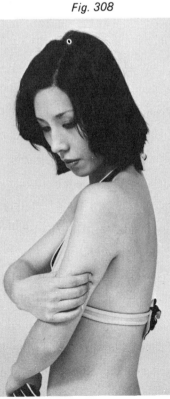

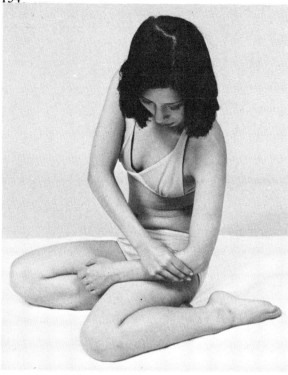

Fig. 309

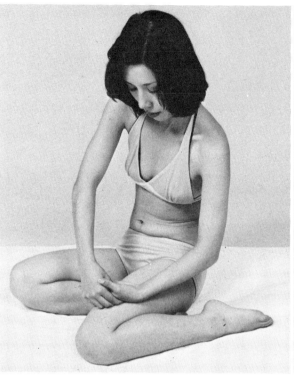

Fig. 310

Give gentle shiatsu by squeezing the arm from the shoulder down to the elbow as seen in Fig. 309. Place your thumb on the inside of your arm with your four fingers resting on the outside. Press with your thumb and squeeze the outside of your arm with your fingers. For a toothache in the upper teeth area, apply strong pressure to the heart and small intestine meridians on the outside of the arm (side of the little finger). For toothaches in the lower teeth area, give strong pressure on the thumb (lung and large intestine meridians).

Shiatsu to Prevent Constipation

If you have a gum problem, apply firm pressure along the center line of the inner arm (triple heater and heart constrictor meridians). People with a constipation problem should apply shiatsu in between the thumb and index finger (lung and large intestine meridians) on LI-4 (Fig. 310).

How to Relieve Tension in the Arm

In cases of nervous fatigue, give shiatsu to the center line of the lower arm (Fig. 311). This relieves tension. In order to relieve stiffness in the lower arm, place your arm on the floor under your knee with one hand holding the wrist (Fig. 312). Apply pressure with your knee. Repeat on the other side of the arm (Fig. 313). You can give strong or soft pressure depending on how you use your knee.

Correction of Wrist Dislocation

Energy stagnates very easily at the wrists and dislocation of the joint is frequent. In this case, place your knee on your wrist with one hand on top of the other and lean on your knee.

Spread your fingers apart and hook them (Fig. 314). Pinch and pull your thumb with two fingers (Fig. 315).

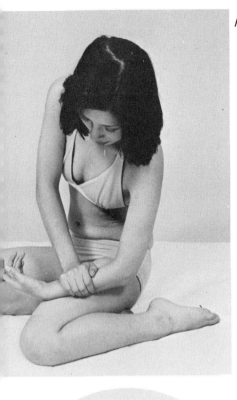

Fig. 311

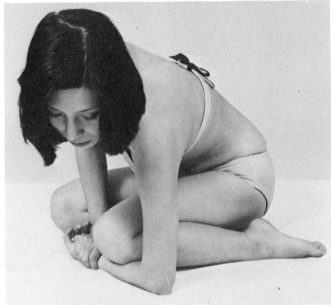

Fig. 312

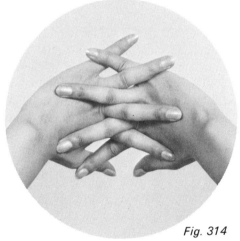

Fig. 314

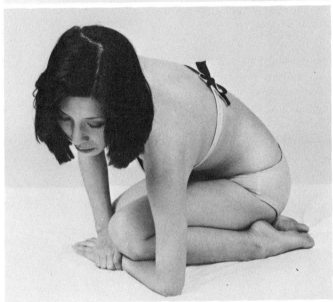

Fig. 313

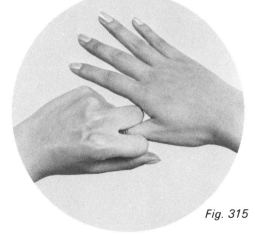

Fig. 315

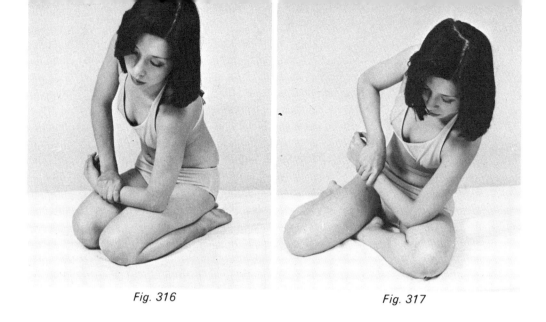

Fig. 316   Fig. 317

Self-shiatsu on the Legs: Sit down in the Japanese style position and place your elbow on the center of the thigh. Give elbow shiatsu (Fig. 316). You can also sit down with your legs crossed or sitting to one side as in Fig. 317. Give shiatsu with your elbow or both hands to the inside of the leg.

Fig. 318

Fig. 319

Fig. 320

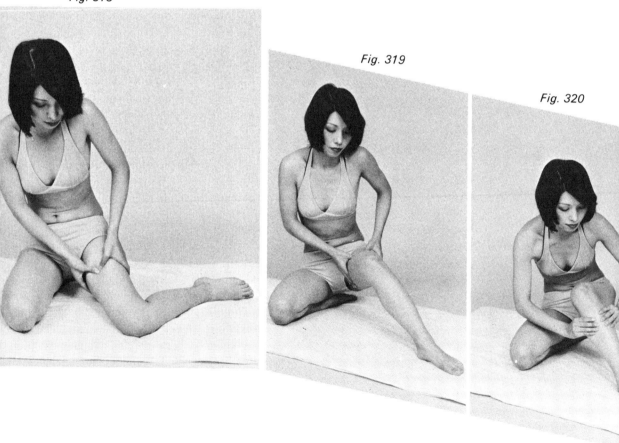

You can bend your legs outward and give shiatsu in the same way (Fig. 318). You can stretch your leg to the side and give thumb shiatsu to the top of the thigh (Fig. 319). Place your thumbs together on the calf muscle with your four fingers from each hand resting on the side of the shinbone and squeeze (Fig. 320). In cases of calf spasms, apply more pressure to the calf area.

How to Stop Numbness in the Calf When your leg is numb due to abnormal circumstances such as after a long sickness, give strong shiatsu from ST-36 on the frontside of the shinbone to the ankle on the outer side of the leg (Fig. 321).

Give shiatsu to the toes individually. Bend your toes and give shiatsu with either your thumb or fingers to the soles and ankles (Fig. 322). Then give shiatsu to the ankle area. Rotate your foot. In Japan this technique is good for longevity and rejuvenation. It is also good for cerebral hemorrhage, stiffness in the ankle and toe area, and difficulty in mobility in rotating the leg. Bruises and dizziness are symptoms of stiff soles in the feet.

Sitting in the Japanese style, you can give shiatsu to the toes and soles and prevent numbness in the leg (Fig. 323).

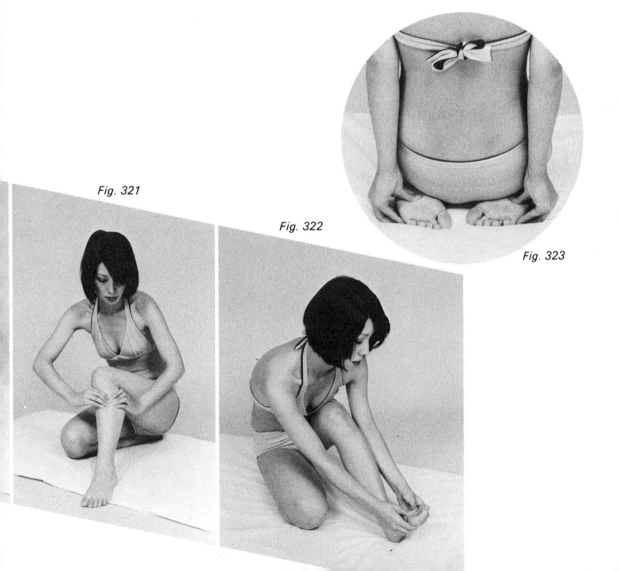

Fig. 321

Fig. 322

Fig. 323

Fig. 324

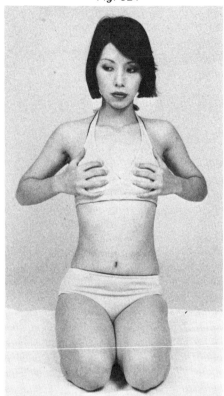

Self-shiatsu on the Chest: When you have a cough or difficulty in breathing, heaviness or pain in the chest area along with mucus discharge, you can give chest shiatsu to yourself. Open your fingers and apply the tips of the fingers in between the rib cage from the side of the rib cage toward the center of the chest (sternum) (Fig. 324). Give pressure and slide upward. Do this to each side. Then with both hands from the center of your chest to the side give shiatsu with your fingers opening and pressing downwards.

Slide your fingers up and down the sternum (Fig. 325).

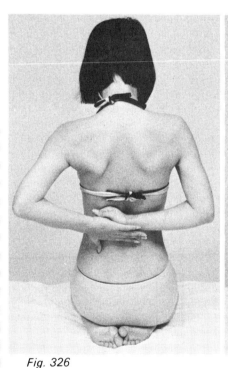

Fig. 326

Fig. 327

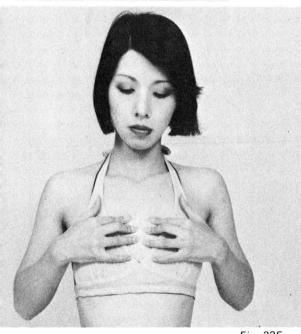

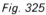

Fig. 325

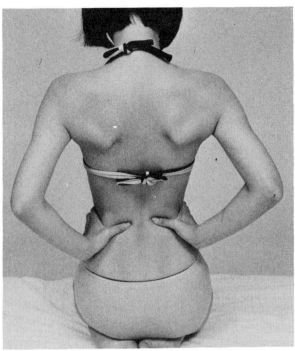

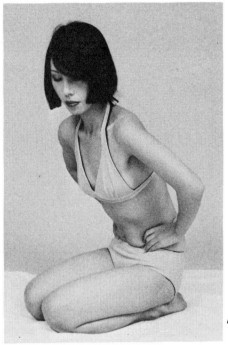

Fig. 329

Fig.328

How to Give Shiatsu to the Lower Back Area: Place your fist on the hara area of your back and apply pressure with the other hand on the top of the fist (Fig. 326). In the curved area of your lower back, place your hands so that the thumb and four fingers rest on the sides of the spine. Squeeze (Fig. 327).

Place your hands on the side of your waist so that the thumbs rest on the lower back area and the four fingers of each hand rest on the large intestine meridian (Fig. 328). Squeeze. An excellent technique for constipation is squeezing your large intestine meridian while evacuating your bowels (Fig. 329).

Self-shiatsu on the Hara Area: Place one hand on the rib cage and support it with the other hand. Press (Fig. 330). Place your four fingers on the solar plexus area and place the other hand on top. Press slowly and softly (Fig. 331).

Fig. 331

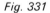

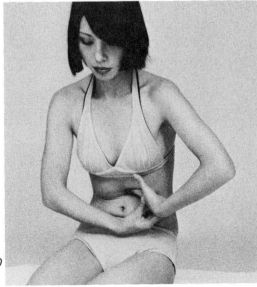

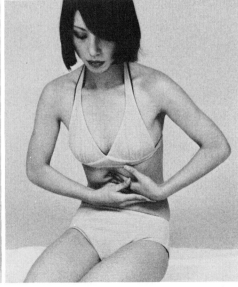

Fig. 330

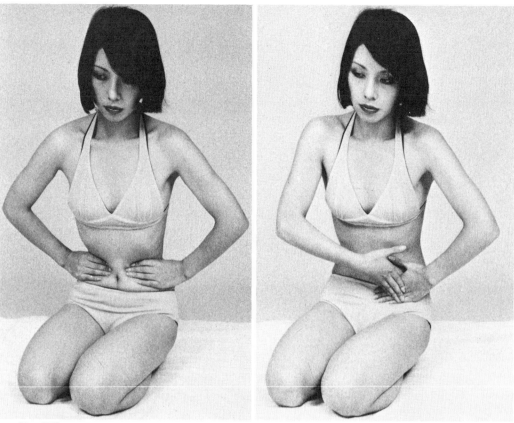

Fig. 332   Fig. 333

Place your four fingers of both hands on the middle of the hara with your thumbs resting on the side. Squeeze (Fig. 332). Put your fingers slightly vertical on your lower torso. Place your other hand on top and press (Fig. 333). When your hands are free, you can give self-shiatsu to the entire hara area. This can stimulate your digestive organs and their functions. This is good for a weak stomach, constipation, and especially no appetite.

Self-shiatsu Lying Down

When you are administering shiatsu, you may get tired making it difficult to continue. The methods in this section can be done when you lie down on either side, front or back by using your own body weight. These methods are very effective and prevent or eliminate fatigue.

Self-shiatsu to the Arm: Lie on your side and give shiatsu from the shoulder to the elbow with the opposite hand (Fig. 334). Don't use your body weight. You can expose your arms more and squeeze it by leaning backwards.

Body Weight on the Arm Place the outer side of your lower arm under your hips and hold. Do not give shiatsu (Fig. 335).

Place the inside of your arm under your hips and hold. You can give holding shiatsu from the elbow to the wrist by changing the angle of your arm (Fig. 336). Repeat on the other side. Lying on your back, place the outside of your lower arm under the hipbone and hold. You can give shiatsu to the arms by using the weight of the sacrum or lumbar vertebrae area (Fig. 337). Repeat with the other arm.

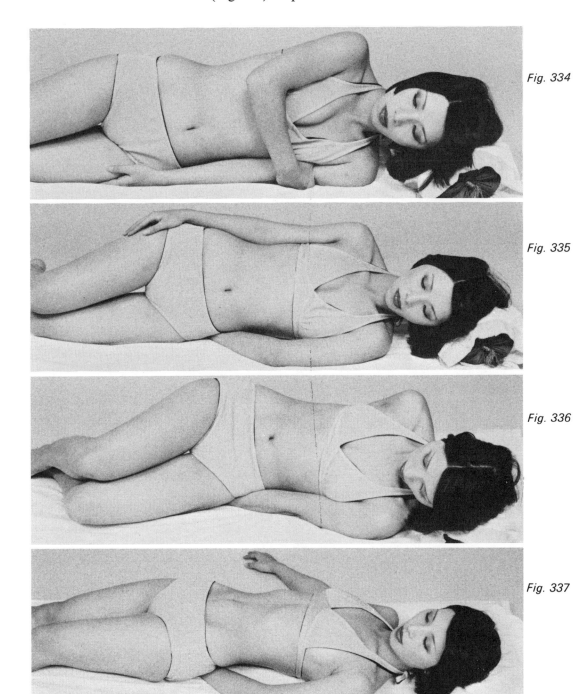

Fig. 334

Fig. 335

Fig. 336

Fig. 337

Self-shiatsu on the Legs in the Supine Position: Lying on your back with one leg stretched, bend the other leg and bring it to the groin area as high as possible on the stretched leg (Fig. 338). You can give shiatsu by sliding the foot of the bent leg down to the kneecap, and from the kneecap down to ST-36 to the ankle along the stomach meridian (Figs. 339–341).

Fig. 338

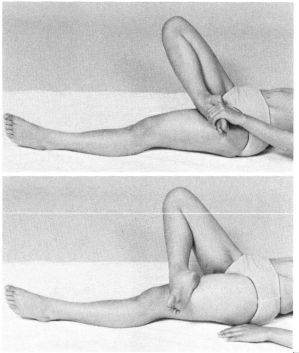

Fig. 342

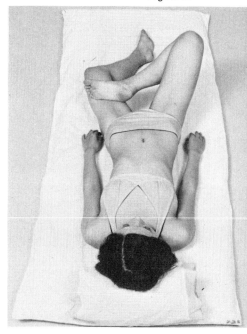

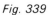

Fig. 339

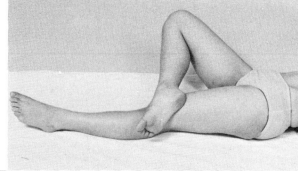

Fig. 340

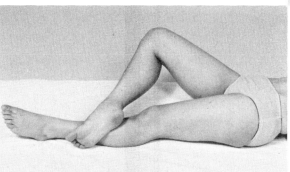

Fig. 341

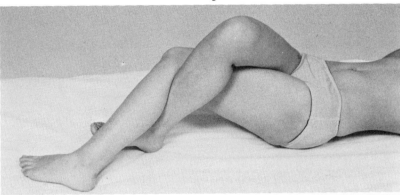

Fig. 344

Fig. 343

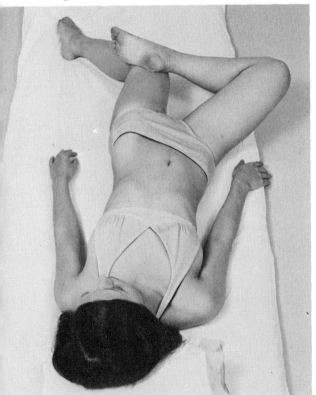

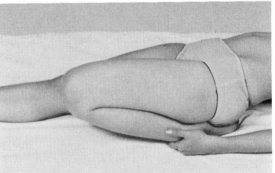

Fig. 345

Shiatsu to the Inside of the Leg	Bend one leg inward and bring the opposite foot as high as possible to the groin area. Press with the foot down the inside of the bent leg from the knee to the ankle (Fig. 342). Turn the bent leg outward and with the opposite foot press down the outside of the leg in the same manner as in Fig. 342 (Fig. 343).
Backside of the Lower Leg	Cross one leg over the other and give shiatsu with your toes to the calf area (Fig. 344).
	First bend one leg and put your toes under your hip (Fig. 345).

Then bring the other leg and do the same (Fig. 346). This technique stretches the stomach meridian. Place your ankle on the opposite knee. Slide down slowly giving continuous pressure toward the floor on the lower leg (Fig. 347).

Fig. 346

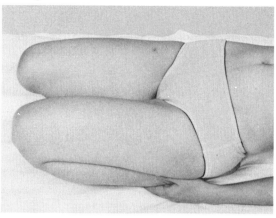

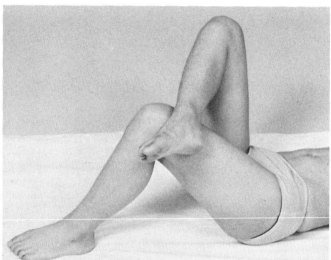

Fig. 347

Fig. 349

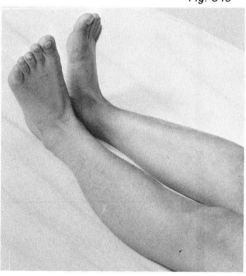

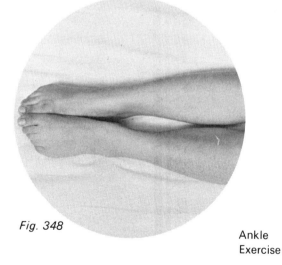

Fig. 348

Ankle Exercise

Stretch both legs and point your toes as hard as possible (Fig. 348).

Flex your toes then point (Fig. 349). Repeat a few times. Then flex and point your toes alternately, keeping your body relaxed. This is good for your tired legs, insomnia, poor digestion, poor appetite, and poor circulation in the legs.

Self-shiatsu to the Lower Back Area in the Supine Position:　Lying on your back, place both fists under your back along the spine. Let your body weight rest on the fists (Fig. 350). Slide your fists from the highest part of the back you can reach down to the hips.

Place a pillow on the lower back area with the palm and fingers of one hand on the pillow (Fig. 351). Rest your body weight on your hand and squeeze the lower back with your fingers and palm. The other hand should support your body at the hips. Do to the opposite side.

Fig. 350

Fig. 351

Fig. 352

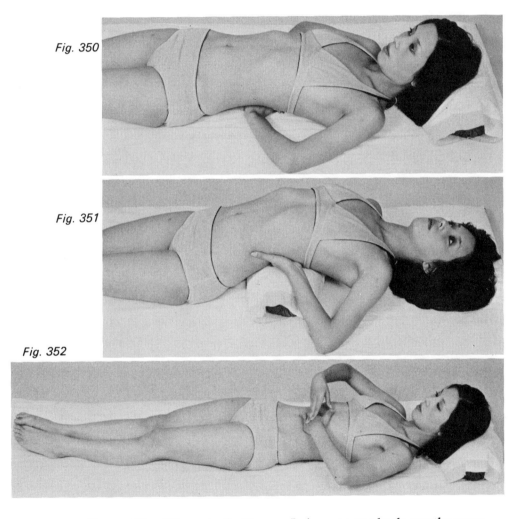

How to Give Shiatsu to the Hara:　Lying on your back, use the same technique for the hara in the sitting position (Fig. 352). Use both hands and feel for any heaviness in the chest and hara area. If you use a blanket or cover on top of your body, the weight of these things will give you efficient pressure.

146

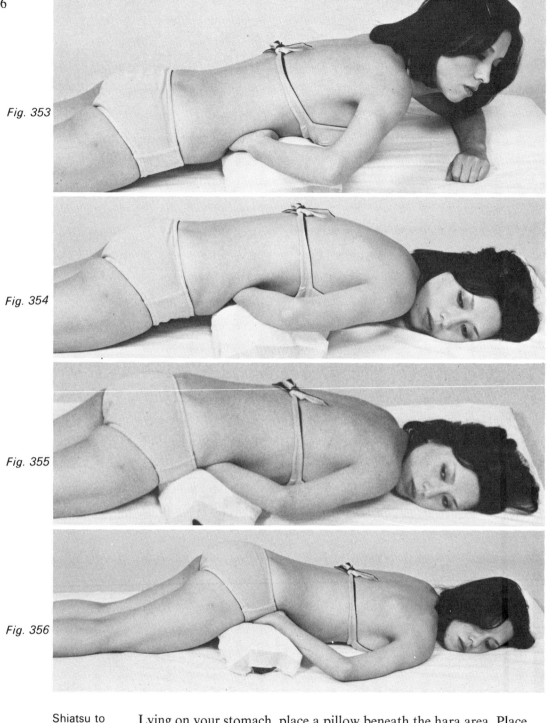

Fig. 353

Fig. 354

Fig. 355

Fig. 356

Shiatsu to the *Hara* in the Prone Position

Lying on your stomach, place a pillow beneath the hara area. Place one hand on top of the pillow and support your body by bending your other hand at the elbow in front of you (Fig. 353). Put your palm, thumb, and fingers on the upper hara area. Make a small, loose fist and apply your pressure.

Navel Area

Make a loose fist with one hand and place it at the navel area so that the heel of the palm rests on the navel (Fig. 354). Straighten the other hand that is supporting your body. Let your chest lie flat on the floor and turn your head to either side. Hold. Repeat to the other side of the hara.

Lower *Hara* Area Do the lower hara area as in Fig. 353 or Fig. 354. Place your pillow on the area where you are giving shiatsu (Fig. 355). The pillow must be hard. If you use a cushion, bend it in half to make it harder.

Groin Area Give shiatsu to the groin as you did in Fig. 354. When you are doing the right side, use the right hand, left side, left hand (Fig.356). This is more comfortable.

Fig. 357 *Fig. 358* *Fig. 359*

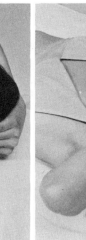
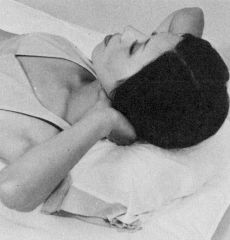
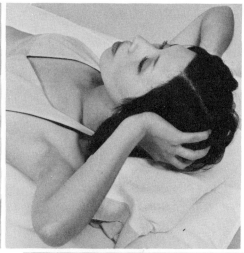

How to Give Self-shiatsu to the Neck and Back of the Head: Lying on your back, put a pillow under your head. With one hand, squeeze the back of your neck. Support your head with the palm of the other hand (Fig. 357). Place your fingers on the cervical vertebrae and give shiatsu from the bottom to the top of the neck. Instead of pressing with your fingers, let the weight of your head sink into your fingers (Fig. 358). With both thumbs, press BL-10, GB-20 area (edge of cranium) (Fig. 359). Then with both palms squeeze your head (Fig. 360).

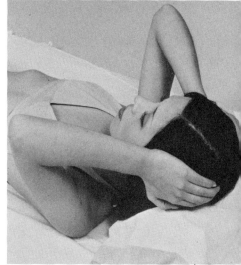

Fig. 360

148

Fig. 361

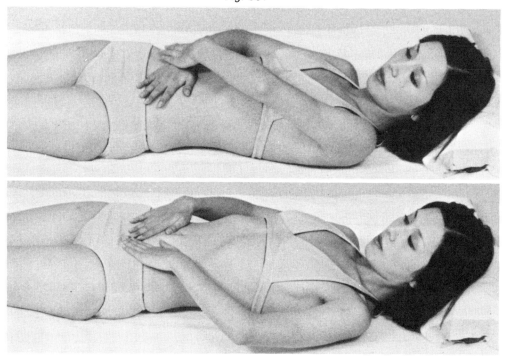

Fig. 362

Summary: You can rub down your face with both thumbs. Rub down your chest, then the hara with both hands. Put your right hand on the navel and apply the location from the left hand by holding the right hand. Open your palms and fingers and put your one hand on the navel area. With help of the other hand, you can give shiatsu by sliding clockwise (Fig. 361).

How to
Breathe

Put both hands on the lower hara area pointing in toward the navel. Calm your breathing (Fig. 362).

Self-shiatsu should be done before you go to bed so you sleep well and wake up refreshed. It is also good for people who are bedridden. It can bring good results and shorten the period of hospitalization.

6. Specific Diseases

Reactions to Shiatsu Treatments

The basic philosophy behind shiatsu is to restore the normal functioning of the body rather than treat symptoms. The longer the body has been neglected and functioning abnormally, the longer it will take to balance itself. During the process of becoming healthy, the body responds to any treatment administered toward this end, but the degree to which it reacts differs in accordance with the type of treatment.

The stronger the treatment or cure that tries to restore the ailing body quickly, the stronger the body reacts to it. Dr. Toudou, a Japanese doctor who employs sedatives in his radical treatments, once stated "Without *Menken* (a reaction), there is no hope for recovery." Though the basic principle behind this is sound, the degree of reaction necessary for recovery does not have to be so pronounced.

When someone is ill, it is natural to seek help that will remedy the situation as soon as possible. Likewise, it is natural for the practitioner to want to cure the patient quickly. However, in trying to do so, we invariably end up treating only the symptoms. Chemical drugs used to anesthetize the pain associated with the symptoms deceives the patient into believing that he is cured.

It is difficult to explain to the patient that the process of recovery is not necessarily entirely painless and symptom-free. Initially strong reactions or prolonged symptoms are often fundamental for proper recovery from an illness. In acupuncture, moxibustion, and Chinese herbal medicine, students are taught and trained to interpret and treat unexpected reactions to therapy. This knowledge is particularly helpful in cases of incorrect diagnosis and treatment. Treatments aim at fast relief usually elicit strong side effects such as drug therapy. In manipulative therapy, however, such danger is usually not present.

The attitude of the patient, on the other hand, is of utmost importance in any treatment. I have treated patients who have gotten worse after a shiatsu treatment and concluded that this type of therapy cannot possibly cure his chronic condition. When a patient asks if shiatsu can cure their problem, I reply that the responsibility for remedying the problem should be placed on the patient himself, not the practitioner. Shiatsu should be a means of allowing a patient to feel himself and realize his healing powers within. It should also be a means of making the patient aware that he made himself sick and therefore should take steps to lead a life style more suitable for his health. The power to cure disease does not lie in super constitutional strength, chemical drugs, or miracles. It is your life force or natural healing power that is the key determinant of whether or not you become and stay healthy. Therefore, in order to become healthy, you should do the opposite of what made you sick.

Alienation and negligence—products of our technological age—have drastically affected our psychological health to the point that sickness and suffering is becoming the preferred way of life. This unconscious desire to remain sick may be a reason why the same treatment given to two different people produces very different results. The practitioner should be aware of those who complain for the sake of complaining. These patients never seem to be satisfied without making one type of complaint or other continuously. Strong criticism is usually aimed at the practitioner. On the other hand, there are people who place the entire responsibility for their well-being on the practitioner. This type of situation in itself is a form of sickness.

It is not wrong to believe that shiatsu can cure all diseases, but you will find that failure will result if the patient's resistance is not broken down. In Japanese, shiatsu is "*te-ate*"—the application of another's hands on the malfunctioning parts of a person's body. These hands take the place of the instinctive desire to place one's own hands on the malfunctioning parts. Thus when you place your hand on the *kyo* point, the patient is able to feel confident about recovering.

When the reaction to a treatment is positive and he feels better immediately after, he is feeling the sensation of total energy which weakens the symptoms present. The symptoms are intensified when they are concentrated in one area rather than scattered throughout the body. In cases where new reactions occur, symptoms that have become chronic are brought back to the acute stage and thus made ready to be expelled from the body.

It is important that you will be sensitive to when your body requires rest, when it is fatigued, in what position it is comfortable, etc. At first, you may notice rapid improvement, but as time goes on, it seems that there is no further changes; you seem to be better, but the symptoms aren't. It must be understood that many stages are involved in recovery and that gaining health is a step-by-step process. It is very similar to the growth of a child. If you are with your child everyday, the measure of growth is more unnoticeable than if you saw the child after a long absence. But whether it is noticeable or not, the fact remains that changes are occurring.

Being aware of this, the professional shiatsu practitioner is patient and understanding. He assures the patient that improvement will come in due time and is sensitive to the needs of his patient during the term of recovery.

Diseases of Locomotion

Sprains: Damage incurred on a ligament or tendon due to sudden or abrupt movement results in a sprain. Twisting an ankle or wrist, whiplash, or chronic tennis elbow can be considered sprains to some degree. Some sprains can be cured easily by massage or application of a heating pad, plaster, or ointments. However, in some cases, partial dislocation takes place. Though it cannot be seen on an X-ray, this type of sprain distorts the muscle and related meridian to such a degree that recovery becomes difficult. Internal distortion caused by external shock greatly affects the internal functioning of the body.

To treat this problem with shiatsu, it is important that you find the distorted meridian lines around the joint area. Place the tonifying hand on the area of pain and feel along the tendon or muscle with the other to find the *kyo* and *jitsu* area. Remember that in order to do this, you must know the meridian lines involved. If you try to sedate the meridian line that is *jitsu*, the patient may find your manipulation too painful. It is better to treat the *kyo* meridians with holding shiatsu, then gradually apply the sedation-tonification technique, stretching the joint area to regain its mobility. In most cases, you will notice more distortion in the *kyo* areas because of the degree of muscle contraction taking place in the *jitsu* meridian. The tonification-sedation technique is fundamental in treating sprains, but it is important that a series of treatments will be undertaken to insure complete recovery. This is even more true in chronic cases.

Whiplash: Traffic accidents are one of the main causes of this problem which affects the cervical vertebrae. Abrupt snapping of the neck forward or backward causing nerve malfunctioning along the head, shoulder, and arms is commonly known as whiplash. Pain in the neck and limited movement in this area can cause headaches, dizziness, ringing in the ears, vomiting, pain in the eyes and throat, numbness in the arms and difficulty in grasping and walking. Treatment by traction, massage, or drugs have not offered complete cures.

In treating such cases, touch the top and sides of the cervical vertebrae one by one very gently. The patient will feel severe abnormal pain in the area of difficulty. Hold his head with your hand so that he cannot move his head suddenly in reaction to the pain. Triple heater and gall bladder meridians are affected not only in cases of whiplash but in any cervical vertebrae problems.

When whiplash occurs, the triple heater meridian is *kyo* and the small intestine meridian *jitsu*. The sudden pull made by the force imposed on it stretches it to such an extent that the small intestine meridian contracts to support the neck. Damage to the cervical vertebrae easily affects the thoracic vertebrae. When the triple heater meridian is involved, the seventh through ninth thoracic vertebrae (heart constrictor meridian area) are affected and often subluxate. Sometimes I find that the small intestine meridian is *kyo* and the triple heater meridian *jitsu*. When questioning the patient as to the details of the whiplash accident, I find that the unexpected thrust came from the side instead of the back or front.

You may find distortion in the area of the first and second lumbar vertebrae which is related to the small intestine meridian. *Kyo* and *jitsu* distortion can also be found in the hara area as well as the legs. Attention must be given to all areas of distortion before good results can be achieved.

In acute cases and at the beginning of the treatment, strong shiatsu should not be employed around the cervical area. Hold the neck firmly but gently so that the patient remains totally relaxed and secure in your hands. Pay close attention to meridian normalization. Chronic cases react well to tonification of the *kyo* area by manipulating the head. Care, however, must be taken by giving a series of total body treatments to prevent the distortion from returning.

Neck Sprain: This condition is usually caused by overstretching the muscle. Maintaining only one position or kind of movement constantly can cause loss of muscle tone and muscle distortion. Gall bladder, triple heater, small intestine, and spleen meridians are affected. General massage is not very effective because it stimulates only the surface. Treatment only in the area of pain is not effective because the problem involves distortion in the internal organ meridians. Since muscle tone is deep, holding shiatsu should be given to the *kyo* areas. Total body shiatsu, using the tonification-sedation technique for the *kyo* and *jitsu* area is important in treating this problem. For further details, please refer to the section on sprains.

Tennis elbow, chronic locomotive malfunctioning, or shoulder pain caused by temporary fatigue require similar treatment. The problem usually does not lie in the area of direct concern but the body as a whole.

Bone Problems: In case of pain and problems of the spine, incorrect shiatsu can aggravate the situation, so it is important that you follow the proper procedure. There are many shiatsu therapists that believe simple pressure to the area of pain cures all. Natural instinct, however, makes it obvious not to press these areas directly. Yet some shiatsu therapists still insist that the patient endure the pain by inflicting more pain, emphasizing that pain cures. Moreover, when the condition worsens, these therapists treat it as a normal reaction to the treatment. In these cases, consideration for total body malfunctioning should be made.

First, gently place your palm on the problem area and then proceed with diagnosis. After diagnosis is completed, tonify the malfunctioning area without applying pressure. If application of the palm to the spine causes pain, this may indicate bone problems or subluxations along the spine.

Give shiatsu to the hara and then check to see if there are any changes in the degree of pain. Total body shiatsu should then be given.

In Japan, we say the bone is the mirror of the kidneys and the spinal column the bladder. Therefore, when bone or spinal problems occur, malfunctioning of the kidneys or bladder may retard the time for recovery. Also malnutrition and poor circulation can cause malfunctioning of the small intestine and triple heater meridians.

Lumbago—Lower Backache: The Japanese have long believed that lower backache is to be expected when you reach 40 years of age. Recently, however, this problem can be found among the 20–30 years age group. The term lower backache is a very general term that can include specific problems such as slipped discs, subluxations of the spine and sciatica. Most lower back problems may be the result of improper bodily movement, bone problems mentioned previously, or internal organ malfunctioning. In order to treat this problem, careful diagnosis is important. In the case of slipped disc, pressing in the area of the problem will not relieve it. The lumbar vertebrae is shaped in such a degree along the hara that often it slips into the dorsal area. This can cause hernia in between the spinal vertebrae, possibly pinching a nerve. It is natural that the lumbar vertebrae respond to the pain by trying to remain erect. This response is also common in cases of whiplash and lumbar subluxations. Most of these types of problems are treated medically with supporters, but shiatsu can also help.

In chiropractic, the subluxated area is adjusted using a thrusting movement. In shiatsu we never press on the subluxated area, but rather try to achieve total flexibility in the lumbar vertebrae area so that the vertebrae return to their normal position.

Shiatsu to the hara improves flexibility and elasticity along the chest muscles as well as corrects any distortions occurring in the lumbar vertebrae region. Find which meridians are *kyo* and work with them in conjunction with hara shiatsu and manipulation by bending and rotating the legs. These techniques relax the distorted muscles that caused any subluxations and allow the vertebrae to move back to its normal position. The specific technique for lumbar subluxations can also be followed. Usually the spleen, small intestine, kidney, bladder, and large intestine meridians are involved.

Stiff Shoulders: Better known in Japan as "frozen shoulders" or a condition marking 50 years of age, there is no specific cause related to this problem. Accumulated fatigue with age, teeth or gum problems causing nerve inflammation and deteriorating internal organ functioning are contributing factors. It is easy to apply pressure to the stiff muscles, but if pain accompanies it, the area may become inflamed especially along the shoulder joint. In this acute stage, rest is preferable to treatment. When conducting meridian diagnosis, you may find the large and small intestine and gall bladder meridians *jitsu*. However, it is more important that you work on the *kyo* meridians. Usually you will find the *kyo* meridians, which are deep and weak, on the opposite side of the pain or *jitsu* areas. *Kyo* meridians are usually the stomach, spleen, heart constrictor, heart, and kidney meridians.

Give holding shiatsu to the *kyo* areas. Do not stimulate the *jitsu* areas. After confirming your diagnosis on the hara and back through the tonification-sedation technique, give gentle manipulation to the arms. Be careful not to overextend the arms in any of the positions you use in the treatment. Forcing the arms into position may give temporary mobility but will increase the pain later on. Through total body shiatsu using the tonification-sedation technique, relief can be offered.

Arthritis: Acute arthritis and rheumatism is often caused by accidents. Chronic tubercular arthritis and gout are accompanied by swelling, locomotive difficulty, fever, and pain resulting in stiffness and contraction along the joint. Dehydration of the joint area gives only temporary relief because it is not part of the natural healing process. Manipulation or stimulation to the joint directly is prohibited. Instead, hold the joint firmly with your palm to protect it and give shiatsu to the meridians and muscles surrounding the joint. This will relax the stiff muscles and tendons and promote better blood circulation to the area. Locomotive difficulty can also be an indication of constitutional lack of energy to move and accummulation of toxins that should be eliminated.

Rheumatoid arthritis and osteoarthritis are characterized by general stiffness in the body with the small intestine meridian *kyo* and the gall bladder meridian *jitsu*. This is often accompanied by difficulties in nutritional absorption in the small intestine, poor circulation, limited locomotive movement, and malfunctioning of our detoxification mechanism. Arthritis in the knee and ankle indicate that the spleen meridian is *kyo*. Sometimes the large intestine, bladder, and kidney meridians are involved. Swelling and puffiness usually affect the triple heater meridian lines.

Rehabilitation: Problems involving locomotive malfunctioning such as a stroke or any type of arthritis often leave the victim only partially cured after medical treatment has been completed. Unfortunately, rehabilitation in this area does not concentrate on correction of internal organ malfunctioning. Instead, the focus is placed on functional and on-the-job training to enable the patient to resume his normal place in society. No attention is paid to the problem the patient still might have with establishing total locomotive freedom and proper internal organ functioning that is necessary for physical and psychological health. Physical therapy is often accompanied with energy revitalization, but correct internal organ functioning is also a prerequisite for total health.

In this area, shiatsu can be of great help in rehabilitating the invalid. By treating the meridians and related organs, total balance, externally as well as internally, can be established enabling the patient to lead a completely normal and healthy life.

Diseases of the Alimentary System

Stomach and Intestinal Problems: When someone has a stomach or intestinal problem, we instinctively rub his back as a gesture of comfort, or have him lie down on his back and gently rub his stomach. The same is true in giving shiatsu. By giving gentle palm shiatsu first to the back, we can arrive at a general diagnosis of the person's condition. After he is more relaxed, confirm the diagnosis by applying shiatsu to the hara area.

Because many problems in this area cannot be named as specific diseases, I have taken the liberty of using common descriptions of each condition along with suggestive indications of how to deal with these problems to obtain quick recovery using the meridian theory. Before reading this section, it is important that you know the twelve meridians concept as well as the method for using *kyo* and *jitsu*.

Nervous inflammation of the stomach—stomach meridian: *jitsu*, bladder meridian: *kyo*.

Overeating, hypertension, gastric hyperacidity, bitterness in the mouth, and perpetual fatigue—stomach meridian: *kyo*, kidney meridian: *jitsu*.

Bloated stomach or overeating feeling—stomach meridian: *jitsu*, kidney meridian: *kyo*.

Intestinal malfunctioning, poor appetite due to lack of exercise—stomach meridian: *kyo*, small intestine meridian: *jitsu*.

Overconsumption of sweets and in-between-meal snacks—stomach meridian: *jitsu*, small intestine meridian: *kyo*.

Abnormal desire to eat—spleen meridian: *kyo*, small intestine meridian: *jitsu*.

Poor digestion due to mental strain—spleen meridian: *jitsu*, small intestine meridian: *kyo*.

Duodenal ulcers—heart constrictor meridian: *kyo*, bladder meridian: *jitsu* or gall bladder meridian: *kyo*, bladder meridian: *jitsu*.

Diarrhea due to overeating—stomach meridian: *jitsu*, large intestine meridian: *kyo*.

Diarrhea from eating too quickly—spleen meridian: *jitsu*, large intestine meridian: *kyo*.

Diarrhea due to cold or shock causing absorption difficulties—small intestine meridian: *jitsu*, large intestine meridian: *kyo*.

Diarrhea due to nervousness—bladder meridian: *jitsu*, large intestine meridian: *kyo*.

Early stage of appendicitis—stomach meridian: *jitsu*, small intestine meridian: *kyo*.

Pus formation—triple heater meridian: *jitsu*, small intestine meridian: *kyo*.

Lack of exercise—triple heater meridian: *jitsu*, small intestine meridian: *kyo*.

Poor digestion due to lack of exercise—small intestine meridian: *jitsu*, large intestine meridian: *kyo*.

Fatigue and lack of endurance due to poor nutrition—gall bladder meridian: *jitsu*, small intestine meridian: *kyo*.

Stomach spasm due to anxiety—stomach meridian: *kyo*, heart meridian: *jitsu*.

Poor digestion—stomach meridian: *kyo*, small intestine meridian: *jitsu*.

For an example on how to treat one of these cases, let us take a case of stomach spasm. You can give shiatsu to HT-5 in your forearm to relieve pain while giving holding shiatsu to the stomach to stop the spasm.

Hernia: There are two major kinds of hernia. One type is inguinal hernia where the contents of the abdomen pass through the inguinal opening or canal in the groin. The other type is umbilical hernia which occurs at the navel. The meridians associated with the internal organs in the area of the hernia are usually *kyo*. The small intestine, large intestine, and occasionally spleen meridians are usually *kyo*.

To treat hernia conditions, support the ruptured area with your palm which in itself tonifies the area. Shiatsu should be given to strengthen and improve the flexibility of the stomach and intestines and to relax the leg muscles and related meridians.

Hemorrhoids: There are many stages of hemorrhoids but the most commonly known one involves the anal area. The Japanese are generally shy about revealing this problem when it occurs, thus aggravating the condition with anxiety.

General shiatsu can improve anal blood circulation and relieve any stagnation of energy in that area by relaxing the muscles of the colon. GV-20 (*Hyakue*) located on the top of the head is very effective in relieving hemorrhoidal conditions. The bladder meridian is effective in treating anal problems and poor circulation. Since constipation is often related to this problem, the large intestine meridian, especially in the leg, should be treated. Care should be taken to avoid excessive drinking and intake of acidic foods because of their adverse affect on the liver and kidney meridians. Occasionally I have had cases where hemorrhoids were related to some mental disorder. In these cases, the heart and spleen meridians were affected and had to be treated.

Liver Problems: In oriental medicine, there is a belief that everything comes from the liver and kidney. It isn't until recently that western medicine has considered the importance of these two so-called silent organs because malfunctioning of these organs usually goes largely unnoticed. When malfunctioning of these organs reaches the pathological stage, it is often very difficult to cure in spite of our current analytical approach toward disease and technologically advanced equipment. Therefore, other antipathological methods should be employed to detoxify the organs.

Oriental medicine focuses on these organs in their treatments with good results. The liver and gall bladder meridians govern and control the total life energy as well as cultivate resistance to disease. Treatment of the liver and gall bladder meridians can be an effective way to balance the body's energy as a whole. Chinese herbal medicine, acupuncture, and shiatsu have helped solve many liver problems when applied before the condition is beyond hope. By treating these two meridians, normalization takes place in problems of congestion, digestive malfunctioning, acute muscle contraction, stiff joints, fatigue, insomnia, and tired eyes.

Liver malfunctioning, according to the meridian theory, indicates that the kidney and small intestine meridians must be tonified or sedated to revitalize the liver. It is also indicative of blood toxification and poor circulation in the heart constrictor and triple heater meridians. By manipulating the joints, you can improve blood circulation, relieve stiffness in those areas and consequently normalize the functioning of the liver. Minimizing your calorie intake and resting as often advised by western doctors, is not as effective as total body shiatsu and joint manipulation.

Gallstones: Bile produced by the liver is stored in the gall bladder sac until it is necessary that it be secreted it into the duodenum. When the bile, through some abnormal chemical reaction, hardens into tiny masses, gallstones are formed. When the stones are in the sac, there is no pain. However, when the stones travel through the bile duct into the duodenum, the walls of the tubes are irritated causing pain near the right rib cage and solar plexus area. Occasionally the pain may travel to the right shoulder and arm as well as cause general stomach upset and congestion. Pain or spasms in the gall bladder may not be an indication of gallstones, so it is important that you diagnose carefully to determine the real problem. When the gallstones are small, there may not be any noticeable pain, but it can be the cause of jaundice, gall bladder and liver inflammations.

The diagnostic points for gallstones are the top of the eighth to eleventh thoracic vertebrae, side of the eighth to tenth thoracic vertebrae, and right side of the tenth to twelfth thoracic vertebrae as well as the right side of the psoas muscle. Diagnostic points for the liver and gall bladder must be used for both diagnosis and treatment.

When the gallstone passes through the gall bladder irritating its walls, the gall bladder contracts causing severe pain. When giving shiatsu, hold this area (the gall bladder) to relax the organ's muscles so that the stones can pass through the tube. From experience, I have found that relatively large stones can pass through easily without much pain. Gall bladder cramp caused by nervous tension or emotional upset can also be treated with holding shiatsu on the entire gall bladder area. The stomach and spleen meridians may also be involved in gallstones becuase of stagnated bile and malfunctioning of the digestive fluids. In cases of nervous tension, check the gall bladder meridian and also the kidney meridian for blood acidosis. In administering shiatsu, it is important to know which meridians are *kyo*.

Diseases of Circulatory and Respiratory Organs

Cardiac Hypertension: Obsessive anxiety due to ignorance of how the heart functions and belief that your heart is your life has led to this problem which I call "civilization disease." The heart has been noted to be the central expression of our total body and therefore responds to any kind of nervousness or stiffness in the spine. Stress often produces stiffness in the shoulders and autonomic system resulting in the bladder meridian being *jitsu*. Subluxations in the heart and heart constrictor meridians areas of the spine can result in a curvature in the thoracic area and increase sensitivity to heart disease. Tightness in the forearms indicates malfunctioning in the triple heater meridian. Check the heart and heart constrictor meridians as well as triple heater meridians in the hara and chest area. In case of palpitations, give holding shiatsu to the solar plexus area and press down toward the navel. For heart pains give holding shiatsu to the stomach area and press downward.

Angina Pectoralis: Angina pectoralis or spasm in the coronary artery is characterized by depression, heavniness around the chest, and fear of death. Complete rest helps in some cases. Myocardiac infraction is caused by deterioration of the myocardium due to blood stagnation in the coronary artery. In some cases it is fatal. A shot of pain is usually felt from the chest and left shoulder to the little finger which involves the heart and small intestine meridians. Before an attack, the patient's heart meridian is *kyo*, small intestine meridian *jitsu*, which can also imply that emotional tension and mental or physical fatigue rather than cardiac abnormality is the real cause of the problem.

Give shiatsu to the liver and kidney meridians for blood circulation, bladder meridian for correcting any autonomic nervous malfunctioning and spleen meridian for poor digestion and lack of oxygen. In case of an attack, give shiatsu to the upper and lower arms, then the back and hara areas. Give steady holding shiatsu and avoid strong stimulative or thrusting movements. If strong palpitations, low body temperature, lack of urine, and pain in the chest area and other signs of a weak heart persist after an attack, consult a doctor.

High Blood Pressure: In Japan, only 10% of all high blood pressure cases lead to a stroke. Therefore, instead of worrying about possible heart problems, we should interpret this condition as a warning that our life style is not compatible with our health. Care should be taken with regard to diet, degree of emotional, mental and physical fatigue, and lack of exercise.

High blood pressure is usually characterized by the heart constrictor meridian being either *jitsu* or *kyo*. When the heart constrictor meridian is *kyo*, the pressure changes rapidly. Hypertension is a common cause of high blood pressure, so administering medicine to patients with this problem does little to solve the problem other than produce side effects. The kidney, bladder, liver and gall bladder meridians often seem to merge together. Little energy is felt in the small and large intestine meridians.

Anemia: Strong palpitations, shortness of breath, fatigue even after rest, poor complexion and lack of vitality are characteristic of anemia. A decrease in red blood cells prevents the proper amount of oxygen from reaching the entire body. Poor diet, hemorrhages, lack of blood, worms and lack of peptic acid and gastric anemia may also lead to anemia. Gastric and intestinal malfunctioning due to fasting for weight loss or an unbalanced diet may result in a mild case of anemia that progressively gets worse. Feeling faint after standing for a long time may indicate brain anemia. People who tire easily or develop skin rashes are easily predisposed to sickness and anemia.

Low Blood Pressure: When our blood pressure surpasses our age plus 90 (systolic pressure), we worry about high blood pressure and heart disease and immediately try to remedy the situation. Because of the emphasis placed on the dangers of high blood pressure, many people associate low blood pressure with longevity and a sign of a healthy cardiovascular system.

The standard rule used to determine whether one's blood pressure is normal is age plus 90. Since this only suggests the average, however, ten or twenty points above or below can still be considered normal depending on the individual. So no matter how old you are, if your blood pressure reading is 120, you can be happy knowing that your cardiovascular system still maintains the condition of a thirty year old.

On the other hand, if the systolic pressure is below 90 and the diastolic pressure below 60, you have constitutional low blood pressure. Fatigue, dizziness, tired eyes, insomnia, headaches, palpitations, shortness of breath, poor circulation, and no appetite, chest and stomach irritability and lack of concentration can all stem from this condition. So when you are treating someone with one or more of these symptoms, low blood pressure may be the cause. Taking drugs or consuming alcoholic beverages to raise the blood pressure will only bring on opportunities for softening of the brain, stomach ulcers, and asthma.

It is essential to lead a regulated life of exercise, rest, consumption of more vegetables and vegetable fat along with total body shiatsu to insure proper functioning of the internal organs. Lack of sleep, smoking, and indigestion should be avoided.

In treating this problem with shiatsu, the following meridians should be considered: small intestine, heart constrictor, triple heater, bladder, and stomach meridians.

People suffering from chronic anemia, poor nutrition, and poor circulation and whose blood pressure is less than 100mmhg (systolic pressure) are usually considered lower blood pressure cases. Though they may live longer than those with high blood pressure, they experience difficulty in sleeping, dizziness when awake, sluggishness, fatigue, and heaviness from lack of sleep. They have a tendency toward autonomic nervous breakdowns, stomach ulcers, and asthma. Lack of gastric acid, stagnation of bile and malfunctioning of the red blood cells cause the stomach meridian to be *kyo*, gall bladder meridian *jitsu*. Improper nutritional absorption and blood regurgitation affect the small intestine meridian while the psychological aspect causes malfunctioning of the heart, bladder, and occasionally liver and kidney meridians. In cases of poor circulation, *kyo* meridians will be heart constrictor and triple heater meridians. Malfunctioning of the triple heater meridian often produces general stiffness in the entire body rendering itself in claustrophobic and suspicious feelings as well as being satisfied with nothing short of perfection. In people who lack sleep or still feel sleepy after a long rest and allergic people with weak skin you will find the kidney meridian *jitsu*, triple heater meridian *kyo*. Allergies and poor circulation indicate bladder meridian *jitsu*, triple heater meridian *kyo*. Total exhaustion, overwork, or tendencies to feel hot indicate heart constrictor meridian *kyo*, kidney meridian *jitsu*.

Coughing: People usually associate coughing with the flu or some respiratory malfunctioning, but according to one classic book on oriental medicine, this phenomenon is related to a variety of meridians, depending on the cause. The practitioner must be well informed about meridian therapy. Choking in the throat and constant coughing are often symptoms of neurotic tension. So-called "cardiac coughing," these same symptoms occur in patients who carry anxieties about cancer. Coughing that produces severe pain along the side of the torso pressing the diaphragm upward can be caused by malfunctioning of the liver produced by overconsumption of high calorie foods, especially sweets (common among children), excessive drinking and exhaustion. Coughing with mucus irritation in the throat may be indicative of malfunctioning of the gall bladder meridian and detoxification process. Among children coughing may occur due to overeating or indigestion. Rest seems to cure the problem but in more serious instances, the cough resumes when the child is active or nettle rash develops. In these cases, the stomach meridian will be *kyo*, kidney meridian *jitsu* or vice versa. If there is stiffness in the back area due to coughing from hypertension, check the kidney and bladder meridians. Pain in the arm, especially the thumb, toward the chest may indicate lung and large intestine meridians malfunctioning. In cases where worms are the cause for coughing, the stomach meridian should be checked for proper functioning. Check the triple heater meridian in cases where the patient is susceptible to tonsillitis, sore throat, bronchitis and colds. Nasal congestion or difficulty in smelling indicates large intestine and bladder meridians malfunctioning.

Problems of the Nervous System

Infant Paralysis: Malfunctioning of the central nervous system, apoplexy, polio, coldness in the extremities, rheumatoid arthritis, neuritis and beriberi can cause paralysis. It is often accompanied by a high fever, pain and numbness or muscle contractions. Facial paralysis, a common problem, is characterized by no expression, difficulty in closing the eyelids and mouth, inability to whistle or swallow effectively, uncontrolled salivation and tearing. In addition, nerve paralysis may occur in the region of the thighs and lower legs. Neuralgia or neuritis may attack the shoulder and scapula, chest, and back areas, impairing locomotive functioning.

In treating paralysis, check for any curvature or subluxations in the lumbar, thoracic and cervical vertebrae as well as the sacrum. Also check the joint areas in the shoulders, elbows, wrists, legs, hips, knees and ankles.

Because you cannot always find *kyo* and *jitsu* in the area of the problem, hold the area in question while checking where the distortion really exists. You can do this by diagnosing the associated muscle and joint area. You will find that the distortion will change from a superficial phenomenon to a deeper one and will constantly be changing. Therefore it is important that you check this before each treatment.

Neurosis: Because of the difficulty of attributing this problem to a specific physical phenomenon, doctors dismiss this as a psychological problem based on imaginary discomfort. Not much attention was paid to this problem in the past but now doctors are freely prescribing drugs to alleviate the problem. About one-third of all chemical drugs are prescribed for autonomic nervous neurosis or psychological anxiety. These poisons, in the form of tranquilizers, are given with the belief that the patient will be cured. A great fault of western medicine is that they cannot effectively treat problems that cannot be placed under a specific category.

In shiatsu we believe that the patient really is suffering from mental and physical discomfort and treat it accordingly. In cases of autonomic nervous tension, the bladder meridian is affected; anxiety and obsession with fear involves the kidney meridian; the stomach meridian is connected with digestive neurosis and anxiety; spleen meridian for over-thinking; heart meridian for impatience; small intestine meridian for poor circulation; gall bladder meridian for headache and eye pain; lack of drive and exhaustion is related to the liver meridian; heart constrictor meridian for palpitations, and triple heater meridian for heaviness in the head and eye pain. In cases of hysteria, tight stiffness in the solar plexus occurs with the heart meridian being *jitsu*.

This dichotomy between the psychological and physical aspect of the patient places the western doctor at a disadvantage. In oriental medicine we combine these two aspects because we believe that one affects the other and vice versa. Because of our total approach to human disease, sickness becomes a complicated problem involving many different aspects but something that can be treated effectively.

Problems of Metabolism and the Endocrine System

Diabetes: Due to lack of insulin from the islets of Langerhans in the pancreas, blood sugar is not well consumed in the cell, thus accumulating abnormally. Sugar present in the urine indicates diabetes. Treatment of this disease usually involves lowering of the blood sugar with the aid of drugs like insulin. However this type of treatment only cures the symptom but not the cause. In many cases diabetes, or hypertension, involves not only the pancreas but also the kidney. Basedow's disease or other side reactions are often experienced with the intake of insuline drugs. Because the problem of diabetes caused by malfunctioning of the Islet's of Langerhans has not been solved, insulin drugs only act as a treatment for symptoms of excessive blood sugar. People suffering from diabetes eliminate sugar in the urine and are always thirsty, with a tendency to overeat, especially sweet foods. Perpetual fatigue, a decrease in sexual vitality, itchy feeling on the skin, neuralgia, numbness, high blood pressure, arteriosclerosis, cataract and poor eyesight are also characteristics of diabetes. It is interesting to note that these problems sometimes occur as a reaction from insulin drugs. People who have a tendency to overeat, are nervous and lack exercise and use their nerves and brain in excess are prone to diabetes. From the meridian point of view, diabetes is characterized by spleen meridian *kyo*. The kidney and bladder meridians should be treated for acidosis and the liver and gall bladder meridians for excessive intake of calories and lack of sexual drive.

Gout: This disease is characterized by severe penetrating pain in the big toes during the night. This pain subsides after one week but occurs again. The joint becomes swollen turning red or purple, occasionally accompanied by fever. It is so painful that you cannot touch it. In some instances the Achilles' tendon and ankle are inflamed. In ancient times gout was called the royal king's disease because it was popular among nobles and peers who enjoyed epicurism. After the Second World War, gout was reported in Japan due to the change in diet. Excessive intake of protein and alcohol creates an excess of uric acid which accumulates in the blood and joints of the arms and legs. Also malfunctioning of the kidney, overwork, or influence of the male sex hormones can be factors in causing gout. The middle aged male is the common victim of this disease.

The spleen and liver meridians are important in the treatment of gout because they are related to the big toe and Achilles' tendon. Attention should also be paid to the kidney and bladder meridians. Shiatsu is most effective in preventing recurrences of this disease.

Basedow's Disease: This common problem among 20–30 years old females involves malfunctioning of the thyroid hormone producing swelling in the area of the Adam's apple, strong and rapid palpitations, protruding eyeballs, unsteady hands and eyelids, nervous excitement and insomnia. The thyroid gland, eye malfunctioning and insomnia belong to the gall bladder meridian lines, while protruding eyeballs relate to GB-31 (*Fushi* point). Tightness in the back and sore throat may be caused by a subluxation in the fourth to sixth cervical vertebrae. The gall bladder and triple heater meridians are *kyo*. Palpitations are related to the heart constrictor meridian lines and nervousness to the kidney and bladder meridians. The triple heater meridian should be treated to relax our arms. The heart constrictor and small intestine meridians are affected by any curvature in the spine and cervical vertebrae and should be adjusted.

Menopause: In many women the cessation of their menstrual cycle brings on many symptoms of malfunctioning. Palpitations, dizziness, excess perspiration, headaches, ringing in the ears, and shoulder pain as well as obesity, perpetual fatigue and mental disorder are often due to hormone imbalance. Because it is often difficult to determine the exact cause for this myriad of problems, the doctor too easily and blindly administers hormone drugs. These drugs, however, only prolong the difficulties involved with menopause. Perpetual fatigue, both mental and physical, poor diet and reactions to operations such as an abortion, indicate serious female malfunctioning.

When the patient experiences dizziness, ringing in the ears and shoulder pain, the small intestine meridian should be considered because of its relation with the functioning of the ovaries. Stomach and nervous disorders or overeating from frustration are related to the spleen and stomach meridians. Palpitations and nervous disorders can be related to the heart, kidney, and bladder meridians. Perpetual fatigue, obesity, headache involve the triple heater meridian while the gall bladder meridian governs hormone imbalance and obesity. It is important that accurate diagnosis be made in treating menopause.

Diseases of Urinogenital Organs

Renal Diseases: There are so many kinds of kidney problems that even the professional doctor finds it difficult to pinpoint. But in shiatsu treatment does not depend upon what category the condition falls into but rather on the phenomena occurring in the meridians in the form of *kyo* and *jitsu*.

In cases of acute kidney problems it is common sense to give strong shiatsu to the kidney area. Poor intake of oxygen and malfunctioning of the detoxication process causing blood pollution is related to kidney nephritis. Lung, large intestine and spleen and stomach meridians are affected from overeating and indigestion. In the case of nervous disorder, or obsession with the sickness, heart and small intestine meridians are important. Check the heart constrictor and triple heater meridians in cases of swelling, coldness, and high fever or blood pressure. These symptoms can be the cause or result of nephritis.

According to the relationship of the five elements, chronic kidney problems definitely influence the functioning of the liver meridian because of the relationship of water (kidney) to wood (liver). The influence of an unhealthy kidney on the liver and gall bladder meridians can cause poor appetite, perpetual fatigue, and tiredness in the eyes.

Total body shiatsu along with a good diet and improvement in mental stability have given much better results in curing renal diseases than drug therapy. In some cases, where the problem is more fundamental and related to the patient's inherited constitution, more time and patience is required for recovery.

Cystitis: Frequent urination followed by pain, insomnia, nervousness, and pain in the lower back are common symptoms of bladder infections. In the case of pyelitis, high fever and shivering due to chillness are felt. The main cause of most bladder infections is bacillus causing constipation, diarrhea, menstrual irregularity, prostate problems, malfunctioning of the urinary system, and coldness in the lower hara. Usually you will find the small intestine, triple heater, and large intestine meridians *kyo* due to coldness in those meridians while the bladder meridian is *jitsu*. In abnormal mucus secretions, the triple heater meridian is *jitsu*, bladder or kidney meridians *kyo*. Accurate diagnosis can be made by holding the hara area. Lack of exercise influences the spleen and stomach meridians and prostate and other problems relating to the reproductive organs affect the liver and gall bladder meridians.

Prostate Problems: Deterioration of the prostate gland that produces semen causes the gland to swell and press against the urinary tube making urination difficult. To some people, removal of this gland is the only answer. But since this is a complicated step to take, it is worth trying shiatsu first. Even in serious cases, you can achieve relief from pain and uncomfortability with shiatsu. In diagnosing this problem, you will find the liver meridian *kyo* and kidney meridian *jitsu*. With emphasis placed on these two meridians, give total shiatsu to the liver, gall bladder, kidney and bladder meridians using the tonification-sedation technique. In some cases you may have to treat the small intestine, spleen and large intestine meridians.

Impotence: It is quite natural for the normal healthy adult to desire and engage in venereal activity. However, psychological fatigue, hypertension in the autonomic nervous system, and hormone imbalance can adversely affect normal activity. This malfunctioning is termed impotence in the case of the male and frigidity in the female.

There have been many cases where I have administered shiatsu for another reason and cured not only the main problem but also his sexual inadequacy.

Treating sexual problems for its own sake will not produce longlasting results because the problem often relates to more than one thing. There are people whose sexual inadequacy does not stem from any physical malfunctioning. These people are often hypertense, overly enthusiastic with their work and consequently overworked or shouldering to much responsibility.

Emotional factors are usually the cause for frigidity in the female. Sexual embarrassment, restraint for the opposite sex, and association of sex with obscenity are attitudes that contribute to the problem and cannot be ignored. We should all realize that a healthy balanced way of living both physically and mentally, is important in maintaining a happy sex life.

In shiatsu we can diagnose where the problem exists by examining the meridian lines. *Jitsu* in the kidney and bladder meridian lines reveals overstimulation of sexual hormones, making it difficult for emotional relaxation, proper sex drive, and normal hormone functioning. In cases of failure to erect and premature ejaculation, the liver and gall bladder meridians that govern blood circulation are very important. If the spleen meridian is "hard" or tight, as is often the case in diabetes, the patient may be suffering from lack of sex drive. The heart and small intestine meridians are also associated with this problem. Lack of exercise may also be one factor involved with sexual malfunctioning. In this case, the lung and large intestine meridians should be normalized.

Shiatsu can work effectively in establishing a balanced flow of energy in the body that is most conducive for sexual potency. However, the practitioner should be aware that emotional and psychological factors are also involved and play an equally important role in maintaining a balanced energy flow.

Problems of Cutaneous Sensation

Rash and Athlete Worms: Unhealthy skin lacking resistance to environmental bacteria as well as psychological stress are often causes of these problems. Improper elimination and inability to detoxify the body further weaken the body's resistance. The lung and large intestine meridians, both related to the skin, should be normalized to improve the functioning of the skin. Internal poisoning mainly caused by psychological stress affect the small intestine meridian, so this meridian should also be treated. To balance the body, treat the kidney and bladder meridians to control body liquids; liver and gall bladder meridians to detoxify poisons in the blood; spleen and stomach meridians to insure proper functioning of the digestive tract; and triple heater meridian to decrease the effects of psychological stress. Giving total body shiatsu is a natural and effective way to cure these problems without the use of drugs.

Eye Problems: The eye is a very delicate organ that consumes more oxygen than any other organ in the body. The liver and kidney also require very large amounts of oxygen. When there is a lack of oxygen in the body, these three organs compete with each other for their share. The eye is not directly related to the maintenance of life itself as the other two organs so it usually ends up with the oxygen remaining after the liver and kidney requirements are filled. Therefore, when fatigue sets in and the functioning of the liver is altered, the eye is affected also.

In oriental diagnosis, the cornea is related to the liver meridian; the outer and external canthus, tail of the eye to the heart meridian; the edge of the eyelid to the spleen; the white part of the eye to the lung; the pupil to the kidney; and the retina to the triple heater meridian. Viewing the eye from a meridian standpoint, the liver and gall bladder meridians are most important. The kidney and bladder meridians are important for liquid homeostasis and autonomic nervous conditions. The lung and large intestine meridians are responsible for normal functioning of oxygen intake and elimination of toxins. LI-11 brings relief to tired eyes.

Eye problems caused by mental shock affect the heart and small intestine meridians; poor diet and diabetes affect the spleen and stomach meridians; pain or abnormal pressure in the back of the eye affects the heart constrictor and triple heater meridians. Judging from our meridian theory, it is understandable why some people believe the eye is the mirror for the whole body.

Myopic patients can benefit greatly by adhering to a good diet, eating in moderation, and total body shiatsu to relieve shoulder pain and to keep the neck and autonomic nervous system relaxed. You can also give shiatsu around the eyes and on the eye itself using the palm of your hand.

Ear Problems: Some common ear problems are otitis externa which is caused by inflammation of the external ear; tympanitis caused by the flu, swimming, or problems stemming from the nose and throat; ringing in the ear, vomiting, and dizziness

—all caused by malfunctioning of the internal ear or other organs such as the nose, brain, stomach, intestine, and eye. Menopause may also cause an imbalance in the internal ear.

Treating points on the bladder meridian and governing vessel located on the head are very effective in remedying ear problems. Points on the triple heater and gall bladder meridians in the area of the ear as well as the neck and back of the head are effective for headaches and ear problems. The small intestine meridian that is located in the inner ear and the stomach meridian located in the nose are also important. In the case of pain in the ear, treat the lung and heart meridians; for high blood pressure and arteriosclerosis, treat the heart constrictor meridian.

Acupuncture is well-known as an effective method for treating ear difficulties including tympanitis. Since the theory behind shiatsu is based on the same tsubos or points, it can also be an effective way to treat the same problems. Simultaneously, shiatsu can also revitalize the entire body because it deals with the meridian lines and their relationship to the entire body.

Gynecological Problems

Menstrual Irregularity: Malfunctioning of the ovaries causing an abnormal menstrual period with pain before, during, and after the period involves malfunctioning of the stomach and small intestine meridians. Therefore, these meridians are important in treating menstrual problems. Other meridians that may be treated are the heart meridian for proper functioning of the diencephalon and pituitary gland; the bladder meridian for normal functioning of the uterus, and autonomic nervous system; kidney meridian for healthy functioning of the glands, especially those involved with the sex hormone; spleen meridian for elimination of any adverse psychological feelings such as frustration; and triple heater meridian for normal mucus secretion in the uterus. General shiatsu administered to the lumbar vertebrae area, between the third and fifth lumbar vertebrae, as well as the sacrum area also help establish menstrual regularity.

Leucorrhea: Abnormally heavy menstrual discharge accompanied by inflammation and itching in the labial area is termed leucorrhea. Caused by Trichomonous and other viral infections, it also affects the uterus and ovaries often producing inflammation in these areas. Insomnia and nervous outbreaks compound the problem making it difficult to cure by drugs alone. In dealing with female problems in general the small intestine and triple heater meridians are very important. When there is coldness and poor or abnormal circulation in the pubic area as in the case of leucorrhea, treat the large intestine meridian and manipulate the legs to release and prevent stagnation in the region of the pubic bones. To help alleviate nervous tension, give shiatsu to the back of the head and arms.

Pregnancy: During the early stages of pregnancy, hormonal variation and toxins released from the growing fetus cause morning sickness. In a healthy woman, these toxins are detoxified by the liver and eliminated from the body. However, if the liver is not functioning properly, poisons enter the blood and stimulate the nervous system causing emotional and psychologically unfavorable reactions. In many cases, toxins also enter the stomach and cause vomiting and poor appetite. These toxins also affect the kidney causing constipation. Although some doctors recommend abortion in extreme cases of toxemia, these problems can be cured by giving regular shiatsu to the liver, gall bladder, stomach, kidney, and large intestine meridians.

Administering shiatsu during later stages of pregnancy is not dangerous if you avoid strong application directly to the fetus. If you follow my meridian method, you can stimulate and strengthen weak organs in preparation for delivery. For quick and effective relief from pain during delivery, apply shiatsu to the coccyx and sacrum areas. Shiatsu in conjunction with exercise specifically designed for the pregnant woman can prepare the woman both physically and psychologically for an easy and happy delivery.

Lactation Difficulty: It seems ironic to me that inspite of western medicine's efforts to make the breasts bigger and better using various injectional methods and plastic surgery, more women are not able or refuse to breastfeed their children. Overemphasis on beauty rather than purpose is at fault. Recently, however, more women are revaluating and understanding the importance of restoring the breast to its normal function—that of breastfeeding.

Failure to lactate can be caused by underdeveloped or inflamed milk glands, hormone abnormality, improper contraction of the womb, or incorrect nursing habits. Shoulder pain is characteristic to this problem. In the olden days, there were Japanese masseurs who specialized in breast massage before and after delivery of the baby. With the advent of western medicine, however, this speciality disappeared.

To promote lactation and recovery after delivery, it is important that the woman be able to rest in a quiet atmosphere and eat a well-balanced diet. Eating large quantities of food for the sake of lactation will only produce the opposite results.

A very effective and enjoyable method of stimulating the lactate glands can be performed by the husband. Stimulating the breast with some form of affection before and after pregnancy greatly assists in preparing the mother for breastfeeding her child.

When giving shiatsu, gently massage the breasts directly in order to stimulate the lactate glands and relieve any glandular inflammations that may be present. Treat the stomach meridian which passes through the nipples and ovaries as well as the heart constrictor, heart and gall bladder meridians, all of which pass through the breasts.

When the mother is not allowed to rest sufficiently after giving birth, blood can stagnate particularly in the shoulders causing stiffness, headaches, dizziness, fever and mental and emotional imbalance. This same type of blood stagnation occurs in middle-aged women too. You can work on the shoulders and arms to alleviate this stagnation. Giving shiatsu to the bladder, triple heater, small intestine, and gall bladder meridian lines in that area will relax the underlying muscles. To regulate the functioning of the ovaries, to control the internal organs in the pubic area, to purify the liquids in the body and to stabilize the autonomic nervous system, give shiatsu along the kidney and bladder meridians.

Shiatsu for the Infant: One of the most important needs of an infant is for cutaneous stimulation. Infantile disorders such as indigestion, spasm, diarrhea, vomiting, coughing, fever, stomachache, colitis and rash can be easily cured by giving shiatsu to both the back and hara areas.

When an infant is unable to sleep through the night due to overexcitement, fever or upset stomach, apply gentle palm shiatsu simultaneously to the back of the head and hara area.

Unclassified Diseases

Today so many people are becoming victims of ailments for which western medicine has no name. Finally reaching the threshold of tolerance for pain, they decide on which doctor should be consulted. In anticipation of what the doctor will diagnose, worry and anxiety over the possible seriousness of the disease he may have compound the problem. Then the actual visit to the doctor, the full examination and final verdict—nothing is wrong! So they return home with their doctor's advice not to worry while the pain continues.

Modern medicine has made tremendous advancements in curing acute diseases but has paid little attention to the area of chronic diseases that do not place the patient's life in sudden jeopardy but nevertheless still exist. Because of the increase in chronic problems, however, more people are becoming disillusioned with the medical profession and are turning toward folk and oriental medicine that is based on experience and wisdom passed down through the ages. Though the medical profession looks down on folk remedies and oriental therapy as unscientific, they are playing an important role in solving the apparent "mysteries" of modern medical science. Manipulative therapy is probably the best therapy to try first because no preparation is necessary and no side reactions accompany it. Shiatsu can be used safely and effectively this way.

Shoulder Stiffness: There is no other problem so common and difficult to cure than stiffness in the shoulders. For lack of a definite cure, modern medical techniques for treating this problem include vitamin injections, tranquilizers and/or traction or simply a massage or rubdown and a hot bath to promote circulation. Plasters, sprays, massage chairs and vibrators are other popular remedies people refer to when the conventional methods fail.

Some people believe that stiffness comes from the tendons that are located in between the developed muscles while others resign themselves to the idea that this is the price man pays for walking on only two legs in an upright position. In most cases, the fundamental problem lies in internal organ malfunctioning, physical and psychological fatigue or general body distortion.

When administering shiatsu, it is important to diagnose the shoulder area to find

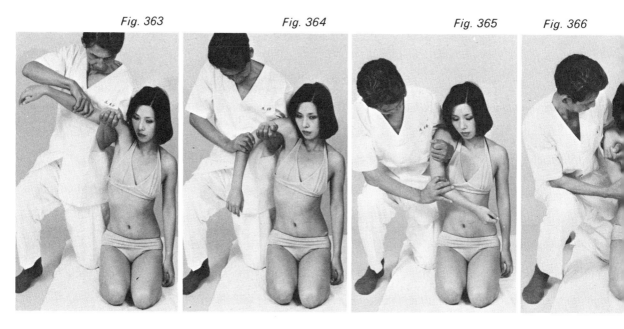

Fig. 363   Fig. 364   Fig. 365   Fig. 366

the basic cause of the problem. Shiatsu given on the shoulder area only will not eliminate this problem. Therefore, it is up to the shiatsu therapist to make the patient understand that his condition is also related to his physical and mental attitude toward life. If successful, the shiatsu therapist will fill the gap that now exists between the doctor and patient in recognizing the patient as a human being.

In treating shoulder stiffness, there are two techniques used. Before learning them, however, it is important that you understand the principle of tonification and sedation of the *kyo* and *jitsu* points.

Have the patient sit Japanese style and place your lower arm under her armpit (Fig. 363). Support her arm at the elbow with the other hand (Fig. 364). Bend her arm at the elbow and bring it towards the front of her body (Fig. 365). Pull up on her shoulder with your arm while pushing her elbow towards the hara. Pull her shoulder up further and press her elbow against her chest (Fig. 366). Rotate her arm and relax it.

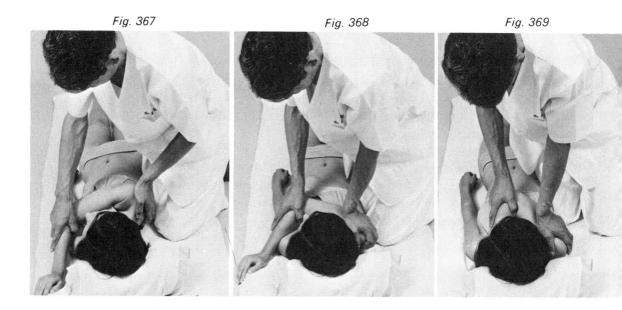

Fig. 367   Fig. 368   Fig. 369

For the second technique have the patient lie on her back. Support her shoulder joint with the palm of one hand. Place her elbow against her chest lifting her shoulder slightly (Fig. 367). Lift her shoulder up towards the chest supporting her elbow against the chest (Fig. 368). Press her shoulder down towards the floor holding the elbow in place (Fig. 369). When the shoulder is on the floor, extend the elbow outward so that

Fig. 370

Fig. 371

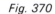

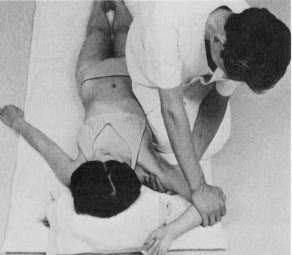
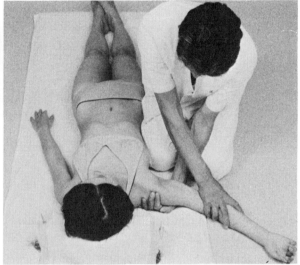

it rests on the floor (Fig. 370). Supporting the shoulder, rotate the shoulder joint with the other hand (Fig. 371).

Hunchback and Curvature in the Back: Though the problem of hunchback in aged people has decreased, perhaps due to the change in life style, curvature in the spine among our younger generation is alarmingly increasing due to an undeveloped hara. In the past parents took it upon themselves to instruct their children to stretch their backs after each meal as well as teach them exercises to maintain proper posture.

Today, reliance on modern medical techniques utilizing the corset and traction as well as injection and hormone therapy with little emphasis on exercise has brought about a generation lacking in a developed hara. Ironically enough in an age where independence and individuality are stressed, how dependent we've become on modern medical procedures to correct problems in the area of health, placing the full responsibility on them and not ourselves.

Chiropractic knowledge regarding curvature of the spinal process asserts that the cause of disease often stems from incorrect alignment of the spine. Correction of this condition is usually rendered by the chiropractor in the form of a chiropractic adjustment. By working on the spine only, a series of chiropractic adjustments are made until the spine stays in place. Little emphasis is placed on the relation between internal organ malfunctioning and the spine. However, working on the spinal column alone covers only one aspect of the problem. In cases of colitis, there is a natural tendency to push the lower spine inward to alleviate the pain, thus causing a distortion in that area due to internal organ malfunctioning. With chest pains, there is often a tendency to stretch the back to alleviate any painful pressure on the chest area. This instinctive form of stretching can be considered an alternative form of treating the spine. In my many years of experience I have often administered shiatsu for some internal disease and unknowingly corrected the patient's chronic spinal condition.

In our clinic, we believe that each spinal vertebra is related to and affects an internal organ, and it is this theory that we base our diagnosis and treatment on. Many believe that because of a subluxated spine curvatures occur in the back. However, we feel that internal organ malfunctioning is the cause for the subluxation to occur. The contraction of the muscles and tendons cause pain that prevents us from instinctively stretching our backs to maintain correct alignment.

Therefore we correct the subluxated area on the spine using the stretching technique, and apply ampuku therapy to the meridians to correct internal organ malfunctioning.

Numbness: Those of you who have studied Zen or another oriental discipline have probably experienced numbness in the legs from sitting Japanese style. This numbness is caused by poor circulation and blockage in the peripheral nervous system in the legs due to tightening of the leg muscles. Standing up becomes difficult too, with the sensation of a sharp tingling pain down the leg and the loss of ability to coordinate your legs. In this case it is important to remain calm and give shiatsu to the *sanri* point (ST-36) and strong shiatsu to the triple heater meridian lines in the leg. As mentioned in the section on self-shiatsu for the legs, stimulate the legs with shiatsu in the sitting position. Generally, people with digestive problems (stomach and intestine) are prone to numbness in the legs. However, chronic and more severe diseases, such as a slipped disc, disc hernia, whiplash, diabetes, arteriosclerosis, brain hemorrhage, pinched nerve, etc. can also be the cause for such numbness. Appropriate treatment should be given for these cases. General numbness indicates abnormal functioning of the nervous system as well as blood circulation, and a high strong nature.

Therefore consistent shiatsu should be given to the center and the extremities of the nerve and blood system. Pain usually appears in the disc point whereas numbness occurs in the *kyo* meridian, in particular the triple heater meridian lines. After diagnosing what is *kyo*, proper shiatsu can be administered.

Muscle Spasms: I'm sure that all of us have experienced a muscle spasm in one form or another. Though we often do not take it seriously, it has caused many a fatal accident. Probably the most common spasm occurs in the calf. It is very common for swimmers who are fatigued or have not warmed up their muscles to experience muscle spasms when they are in the cold water, and what about the times when you woke up in the middle of the night with severe pain in the legs or arms? Diet, weak stomach and intestine and lack of sleep can be an underlying cause for spasms, but no other specific reasons have been cited. Poor circulation in relation to the amount of exercise at a given time may be a factor worth considering. For instance, when you suddenly exert your cold muscles, the muscle contracts into a spasm. To relieve muscle spasms, pull the muscle in opposite directions, one toward the muscle origin and the other toward the muscle insertion. Then give shiatsu by gently squeezing the muscle. If the spasm continues, you can support one end of the muscle and tendon and apply shiatsu directly to the spasmatic area. In cases of spasms in the calf area, give strong shiatsu to the back of the kneecap and bend the big toes in the direction of the head. However, one must not forget that incorporating total body shiatsu in one's daily life is the best way to prevent such spasms from occurring.

Stomatitis: Most frequently found among children and some adults, this problem strikes when you are tired or have overeaten. Pain reduces the appetite and small white spots appear. Tiny white creases radiate from the corners of the mouth, fanning out like a bird's foot. This abnormal condition indicates a disorder in the mucus lining of the stomach. Therefore it is important that the stomach be treated first. Shiatsu should also be given to the arms and legs as well as ampuku to relax the tense muscles, reduce nervousness and compensate for lack of exercise—all major causes of the problem. Oral odor may also be an indication of stomatitis, though in some cases, the odor may be due to improperly maintained teeth.

A Japanese proverb states that the stomach is the root of all diseases, all diseases entering through the mouth. Thus it is important that you uphold a healthy style of living, including shiatsu into your daily program to completely clear up your problem and maintain a healthy state.

In giving shiatsu, you will find that malfunctioning of the triple heater meridian, especially in the arms, may be the cause of this problem.

Palpitations: A tremendous amount of energy is needed in order to maintain proper functioning of our entire body. Your heart was originally constructed to withstand the continuous burden of pumping blood to all parts of your body. Strong palpitations occur when you prepare for each movement. With our concern today about heart disease, palpitations have mistakenly been connected with fatal heart conditions. The correct meaning of palpitations refers to a very normal functioning of the heart.

It is only when we begin worrying about it as a prelude to heart conditions that palpitations become a problem. Acute anxiety not only prolongs palpitations but also adversely affects the functioning of the stomach, bringing on unnecessary stomach diseases as well as shortening one's life span.

Total body shiatsu and ampuku therapy are highly beneficial. Gentle shiatsu on the sides of the solar plexus using the four fingers, calms the patient and normalizes the palpitations. In cases where malfunctioning and deterioration of the internal organs is the cause, total body shiatsu is very important. You will find the heart and stomach meridian *jitsu*, and the heart constrictor meridian *kyo* or *jitsu*.

Shortness of Breath: People conduct their daily lives without worrying about their health until the age of forty when they experience fatigue and shoulder stiffness.

Breathing becomes shallow with the entire body swaying with each breath. Climbing stairs or running at full speed leaves you windless and a reminder that you are getting on in age. When you can no longer reach down and tie your shoe lace because your stomach gets in the way, it is time to stop and think about the alarming situation of your health. Insomnia due to malnutrition, poor complexion inspite of a plump figure, dizziness due to anemia—these are a few indications that it is time to give your body a good cleaning. By resorting to shiatsu rather than medicine, a diagnosis can be made by feeling the areas of stiffness and pain as well as the degree of flexibility in the joints and thus prevent the condition from becoming worse. When we become aware of the fact that our bodies can take wear and tear only for so long and that proper maintenance of the body throughout our life is imperative for good health, old age will no longer be dreaded or used as an excuse for the abuse of one's own body.

Nasal Congestion: There are many different types of nasal congestion. There is acute nasal congestion caused by a cold; chronic nasal congestion whereby inflammation occurs with the slightest bit of stimulation; swollen nasal congestion caused by nasal mucus or malformation of the nasal bone; and empyema where the nasal cavity contains pus.

Changes in weather are also believed to affect not only the nose, but also asthma, tuberculosis, arthritis, and neuralgia. I have heard many times of people who have been cured of their long suffering from sinus problems just by going overseas and changing to another climate. Air pollution is another important factor to consider when treating this disease. If the condition is prolonged, malfunctioning of the brain and lungs as well as poor appetite will follow. Drugs and nasal sprays will temporarily cleanse the nasal passages, but not clear up the problem.

Shiatsu provides the fundamental treatment needed to correct this problem. Emphasis should be placed not only on the nasal area but the kidney, bladder, large intestine and triple heater meridians. Because many people with nasal problems have a tendency to overeat, thus weakening the stomach and intestine, attention should also be directed on the spleen and stomach meridians.

When the body is healthy, natural resistance built up in the body will ward off problems that may arise due to changes in the weather or quality of air.

Authors' Note

It was in a dark room in the Lutheran Church in Hiroshima where I began my English conversation classes twenty years ago. It was taught by an American missionary born in California. Though he did not succeed in converting me into a devout Christian, he certainly taught me how to be a rather bold English speaker. From my experiences with my teacher, I often wondered how two completely different cultures could communicate with each other. How can one culture be transplanted into the soil of another? This is the dilemma in translating one language into another. How accurately and to what extent can we do this?

Though I lecture throughout America on oriental culture, I often find myself frustrated and possessed with an indescribable dissatisfaction. Rather than blaming it on my poor English, I began to realize that the problem was the existence of a cultural gap. And I am still trying to fill it in.

At the beginning of my career in teaching, I felt obligated as an instructor to answer all the questions posed by my students whether I really knew the answer or not. For some reason Americans look for and demand and accept ready answers to everything whether it be from a teacher, book, authority, or the next door neighbor. Unfortunately many beliefs are formulated without thorough understanding on the part of the believers themselves. I feel that there are many questions that have no answers and some that have answers that must come from the student himself. Allowing space to grow with an idea and concept is sometimes more important than the concept itself.

I must admit that accepting this assignment to translate *Zen Shiatsu* from Japanese to English triggered nightmares symbolizing the cultural dilemma I had to face in fulfilling this task. But, like Don Quixote riding a Honda motorcycle for the first time, I mustered up the courage and determination to drive ahead. I only hope I haven't knocked down any fences along the way.

I began translating this book not only because I liked the book and thought it might be of interest to the western world, but also out of a sense of duty to both cultures. I cannot express in words the extent of Sensei Masunaga's genius not only for shiatsu but for a philosophy that relates to all mankind. It would indeed be a shame not to share this with the world.

I admire the dedicated work and determination on the part of the publishers to print this book for western readers at this time. The concepts contained in this book are five years ahead of its time. I had advised that the book be published when Americans will be more familiar with this subject, but the publishers' enthusiasm for the book outweighed any business or financial consideration. This attitude is commendable.

My thanks goes to Ms. Pauline Sasaki who helped correct my translation. I must confess that without her assistance, publication of this book in English would have been difficult.

I would also like to express my gratitude to my wife, Bonnie Ohashi, whose advice as a literary agent and professional editor made this book possible.

Last but not least, I would like to say thanks to you, the reader, who is so willing to learn about our oriental philosophy. I hope that in doing so, you will discover that wisdom is not a matter of East and West but a virtue common to all mankind.

Hoping that *Zen Shiatsu* will contribute toward our health and world peace, I share this knowledge and growing with you. I keep myself and my P. O: Box 1011, New York, N. Y. 10019 open to your letters.

With health and Love,

WATARU OHASHI

In conclusion, I must take the opportunity to make the following comments and acknowledgements. I came to entertain the idea of producing an English-language version of this book when my coauthor, Wataru Ohashi, read the original Japanese-language text (*Shiatsu*, published by Ido no Nihonsha) while he was in New York, became interested in it, and suggested that it be translated.

In the past, books on shiatsu have confined themselves to the most fundamental technical explanations for the sake of beginners and have not dealt with the scholarly, theoretic basis of this therapeutic system. My original Japanese text is directed toward the specialist and includes the medical philosophy on which shiatsu rests. This aspect of the book interested Mr. Ohashi, who came to believe that my work could be of importance in gaining wider understanding for both sophisticated shiatsu and for oriental thought in general.

When he proposed the English-language version of the book, I agreed at once and applied to the publisher Ido no Nihonsha for permission to have the translation made. This company not only gave its consent, but also generously offered the use of the negatives of most of the photographs. I am very grateful to them for their kind cooperation.

SHIZUTO MASUNAGA

Index